IMAT Practice Papers

Volumes One & Two

UniAdmissions

ISBN 978-1-912557-81-3

Published by *RAR Medical Services Limited*
www.uniadmissions.co.it
info@uniadmissions.co.it
Tel: 0208 068 0438

IMAT Practice Papers

8 Full Papers & Solutions

Alex Ochakovski
Rohan Agarwal

UniAdmissions

About the Authors

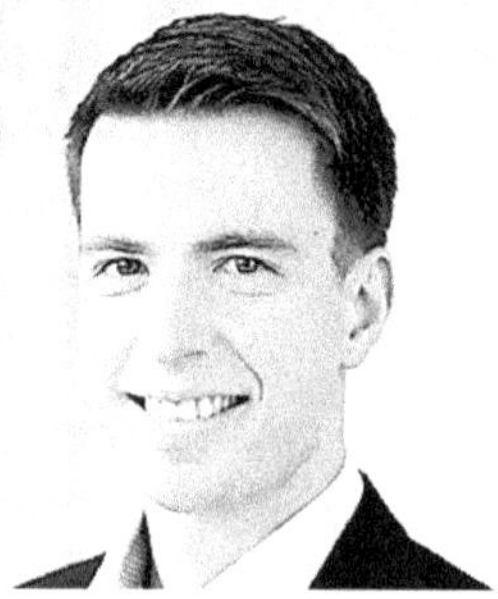

Alex is the co-founder and **Managing Director** at IMAT School, as well as the founder of MEDschool.it website. As a graduate of a first of a kind International Medical School in Italy, a former official supervisor of the IMAT test in Pavia and a dedicated curator of MEDschool.it, Alex has developed a deep understanding of the IMAT and the admission process over the years, following IMAT from the day it was created.

As an avid researcher with over ten peer-reviewed publications, experienced software developer, a fluent speaker of five languages and a medical doctor, Alex feels most fulfilled by combining his passions and strengths in projects that make a positive impact on society.

Thousands of current international medical students have been admitted to medical studies all over Italy with the help of the guidance and resources he provides to this day, creating a country-wide network of contacts in every International Medical School in Italy.

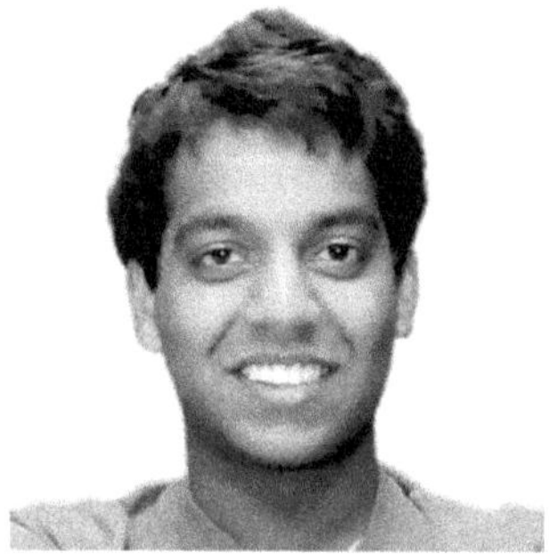

Rohan is the **Director of Operations** at *UniAdmissions* and is responsible for its technical and commercial arms. He graduated from Gonville and Caius College, Cambridge and is a fully qualified doctor. Over the last five years, he has tutored hundreds of successful Oxbridge and Medical applicants. He has also authored twenty books on admissions tests and interviews.

Rohan has taught physiology to undergraduate medical students and interviewed medical school applicants for Cambridge. He has published research on bone physiology and writes education articles for the Independent and Huffington Post. In his spare time, Rohan enjoys playing the piano and table tennis.

INTRODUCTION

The Basics

The International Medical Admissions Test (IMAT) is a 100-minute written exam for students who are applying to read medical and veterinary courses at competitive universities across the world.

It is a highly time pressured exam that forces you to apply knowledge in ways you have never thought about before. In this respect simply remembering solutions taught in class or from past papers is not enough.

However, fear not, despite what people say, you can actually prepare for the IMAT! With a little practice you can train your brain to manipulate and apply learnt methodologies to novel problems with ease. The best way to do this is through exposure to as many past/specimen papers as you can.

Preparing for the IMAT

Before going any further, it's important that you understand the optimal way to prepare for the IMAT. Rather than jumping straight into doing mock papers, it's essential that you start by understanding the components and the theory behind the IMAT by using an IMAT textbook. Once you've finished the non-timed practice questions, you can progress to past IMAT papers. These are freely available online at www.uniadmissions.co.uk/IMAT-past-papers and serve as excellent practice. You're strongly advised to use these in combination with the *IMAT Past Paper Worked Solutions* Book so that you can improve your weaknesses. Finally, once you've exhausted past papers, move onto the mock papers in this book.

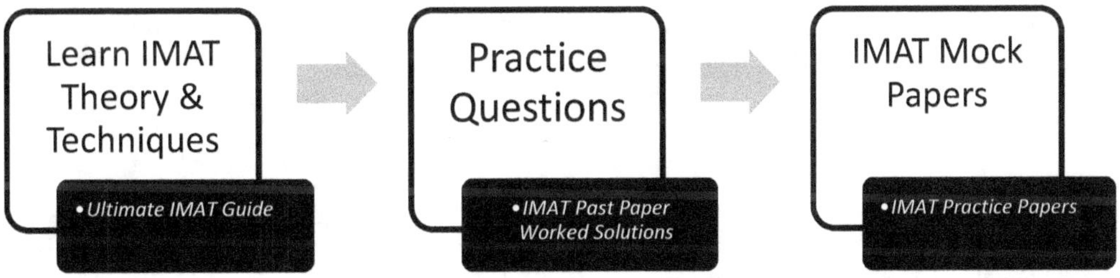

Already seen them all?

So, you've run out of past papers? Well hopefully that is where this book comes in. It contains eight unique mock papers; each compiled by expert IMAT tuors at *UniAdmissions* who scored in the top 10% nationally.

Having successfully gained a place on their course of choice, our tutors are intimately familiar with the IMAT and its associated admission procedures. So, the novel questions presented to you here are of the correct style and difficulty to continue your revision and stretch you to meet the demands of the IMAT.

General Advice

Start Early

It is much easier to prepare if you practice little and often. Start your preparation well in advance; ideally 10 weeks but at the latest within a month. This way you will have plenty of time to complete as many papers as you wish to feel comfortable and won't have to panic and cram just before the test, which is a much less effective and more stressful way to learn. In general, an early start will give you the opportunity to identify the complex issues and work at your own pace.

Prioritise

Some questions in sections can be long and complex – and given the intense time pressure you need to know your limits. It is essential that you don't get stuck with very difficult questions. If a question looks particularly long or complex, mark it for review and move on. You don't want to be caught 5 questions short at the end just because you took more than 3 minutes in answering a challenging multi-step question. If a question is taking too long, choose a sensible answer and move on. Remember that each question carries equal weighting and therefore, you should adjust your timing in accordingly. With practice and discipline, you can get very good at this and learn to maximise your efficiency.

Negative Marking

There is a penalty of -0.4 points for each incorrect answer in the IMAT. This removes the luxury of always being able to guess should you absolutely be not able to figure out the right answer for a question or run behind time. However this does not mean that you should not guess at all. Since each question provides you with 5 possible answers, you have a 20% chance of guessing correctly. Therefore, if you aren't sure (and are running short of time), try to eliminate a couple of answers to increase your chances of getting the question correct. For example, if a question has 5 options and you manage to eliminate 2 options- your chances of getting the question increase from 20% to 33%!

Practice

This is the best way of familiarising yourself with the style of questions and the timing for this section. Although the exam will essentially only test GCSE level knowledge, you are unlikely to be familiar with the style of questions in all sections when you first encounter them. Therefore, you want to be comfortable at using this before you sit the test.

Practising questions will put you at ease and make you more comfortable with the exam. The more comfortable you are, the less you will panic on the test day and the more likely you are to score highly. Initially, work through the questions at your own pace, and spend time carefully reading the questions and looking at any additional data. When it becomes closer to the test, **make sure you practice the questions under exam conditions**.

Past Papers

Official past papers and answers from 2011 onwards are freely available online on our website at www.uniadmissions.co.uk/IMAT-past-papers.

You will undoubtedly get stuck when doing some past paper questions – they are designed to be tricky and the answer schemes don't offer any explanations. Thus, **you're highly advised to acquire a copy of *IMAT Past Paper Worked Solutions*** – a free ebook is available online (see the back of this book for more details).

Repeat Questions

When checking through answers, pay particular attention to questions you have got wrong. If there is a worked answer, look through that carefully until you feel confident that you understand the reasoning, and then repeat the question without help to check that you can do it. If only the answer is given, have another look at the question and try to work out why that answer is correct. This is the best way to learn from your mistakes, and means you are less likely to make similar mistakes when it comes to the test. The same applies for questions which you were unsure of and made an educated guess which was correct, even if you got it right. When working through this book, **make sure you highlight any questions you are unsure of**, this means you know to spend more time looking over them once marked.

No Calculators

You aren't permitted to use calculators in the exam – thus, it is essential that you have strong numerical skills. For instance, you should be able to rapidly convert between percentages, decimals and fractions. You will seldom get questions that would require calculators, but you would be expected to be able to arrive at a sensible estimate. Consider for example:

Estimate 3.962 x 2.322;

3.962 is approximately 4 and 2.323 is approximately 2.33 = 7/3.

Thus, 3.962 x 2.322 $\approx 4 \, x \frac{7}{3} = \frac{28}{3} = 9.33$

Since you will rarely be asked to perform difficult calculations, you can use this as a signpost of if you are tackling a question correctly. For example, when solving a physics question, you end up having to divide 8,079 by 357- this should raise alarm bells as calculations in the IMAT are rarely this difficult.

A word on timing...

"If you had all day to do your exam, you would get 100%. But you don't."
Whilst this isn't completely true, it illustrates a very important point. Once you've practiced and know how to answer the questions, the clock is your biggest enemy. This seemingly obvious statement has one very important consequence. **The way to improve your score is to improve your speed.** There is no magic bullet. But there are a great number of techniques that, with practice, will give you significant time gains, allowing you to answer more questions and score more marks.

Timing is tight throughout – **mastering timing is the first key to success**. Some candidates choose to work as quickly as possible to save up time at the end to check back, but this is generally not the best way to do it. Often questions can have a lot of information in them – each time you start answering a question it takes time to get familiar with the instructions and information. By splitting the question into two sessions (the first run-through and the return-to-check) you double the amount of time you spend on familiarising yourself with the data, as you have to do it twice instead of only once. This costs valuable time. In addition, candidates who do check back may spend 2–3 minutes doing so and yet not make any actual changes. Whilst this can be reassuring, it is a false reassurance as it is unlikely to have a significant effect on your actual score. Therefore, it is usually best to pace yourself very steadily, aiming to spend the same amount of time on each question and finish the final question in a section just as time runs out. This reduces the time spent on re-familiarising with questions and maximises the time spent on the first attempt, gaining more marks.

It is essential that you don't get stuck with the hardest questions – no doubt there will be some. In the time spent answering only one of these you may miss out on answering three easier questions. If a question is taking too long, choose a sensible answer and move on. Never see this as giving up or in any way failing, rather it is the smart way to approach a test with a tight time limit. With practice and discipline, you can get very good at this and learn to maximise your efficiency. It is not about being a hero and aiming for full marks – this is almost impossible and very much unnecessary (even Oxbridge will regard any score higher than 7 as exceptional). It is about maximising your efficiency and gaining the maximum possible number of marks within the time you have.

Use the Options:

Some questions may try to overload you with information. When presented with large tables and data, it's essential you look at the answer options so you can focus your mind. This can allow you to reach the correct answer a lot more quickly. Consider the example below:

The table below shows the results of a study investigating antibiotic resistance in staphylococcus populations. A single staphylococcus bacterium is chosen at random from a similar population. Resistance to any one antibiotic is independent of resistance to others.

Calculate the probability that the bacterium selected will be resistant to all four drugs.

A 1 in 10^6
B 1 in 10^{12}
C 1 in 10^{20}
D 1 in 10^{25}
E 1 in 10^{30}
F 1 in 10^{35}

Antibiotic	Number of Bacteria tested	Number of Resistant Bacteria
Benzyl-penicillin	10^{11}	98
Chloramphenicol	10^9	1200
Metronidazole	10^8	256
Erythromycin	10^5	2

Looking at the options first makes it obvious that there is **no need to calculate exact values**- only in powers of 10. This makes your life a lot easier. If you hadn't noticed this, you might have spent well over 90 seconds trying to calculate the exact value when it wasn't even being asked for.

In other cases, you may actually be able to use the options to arrive at the solution quicker than if you had tried to solve the question as you normally would. Consider the example below:

A region is defined by the two inequalities: $x - y^2 > 1 \; and \; xy > 1$. Which of the following points is in the defined region?

A. (10,3)
B. (10,2)
C. (-10,3)
D. (-10,2)
E. (-10,-3)

Whilst it's possible to solve this question both algebraically or graphically by manipulating the identities, by far **the quickest way is to actually use the options**. Note that options C, D and E violate the second inequality, narrowing down to answer to either A or B. For A: $10 - 3^2 = 1$ and thus this point is on the boundary of the defined region and not actually in the region. Thus the answer is B (as 10-4 = 6 > 1.)

In general, it pays dividends to look at the options briefly and see if they can be help you arrive at the question more quickly. Get into this habit early – it may feel unnatural at first but it's guaranteed to save you time in the long run.

Keywords

If you're stuck on a question; pay particular attention to the options that contain key modifiers like "**always**", "**only**", "**all**" as examiners like using them to test if there are any gaps in your knowledge. E.g. the statement "arteries carry oxygenated blood" would normally be true; "All arteries carry oxygenated blood" would be false because the pulmonary artery carries deoxygenated blood.

Manage your Time:

It is highly likely that you will be juggling your revision alongside your normal school studies. Whilst it is tempting to put your A-levels on the back burner falling behind in your school subjects is not a good idea, don't forget that to meet the conditions of your offer should you get one you will need at least one A*. So, time management is key!

Make sure you set aside a dedicated 90 minutes (and much more once you're closer to the exam) to commit to your revision each day. The key here is not to sacrifice too many of your extracurricular activities, everybody needs some down time, but instead to be efficient. Take a look at our list of top tips for increasing revision efficiency below:

1. Create a comfortable work station
2. Declutter and stay tidy
3. Treat yourself to some nice stationery
4. See if music works for you → if not, find somewhere peaceful and quiet to work
5. Turn off your mobile or at least put it into silent mode
6. Silence social media alerts
7. Keep the TV off and out of sight
8. Stay organised with to do lists and revision timetables – more importantly, stick to them!
9. Keep to your set study times and don't bite off more than you can chew
10. Study while you're commuting
11. Adopt a positive mental attitude
12. Get into a routine
13. Consider forming a study group to focus on the harder exam concepts
14. Plan rest and reward days into your timetable – these are excellent incentive for you to stay on track with your study plans!

Keep Fit & Eat Well:

'A car won't work if you fill it with the wrong fuel' - your body is exactly the same. You cannot hope to perform unless you remain fit and well. The best way to do this is not underestimate the importance of healthy eating. Beige, starchy foods will make you sluggish; instead start the day with a hearty breakfast like porridge. Aim for the recommended 'five a day' intake of fruit/veg and stock up on the oily fish or blueberries – the so called "super foods".

When hitting the books, it's essential to keep your brain hydrated. If you get dehydrated you'll find yourself lethargic and possibly developing a headache, neither of which will do any favours for your revision. Invest in a good water bottle that you know the total volume of and keep sipping through the day. Don't forget that the amount of water you should be aiming to drink varies depending on your mass, so calculate your own personal recommended intake as follows: 30 ml per kg per day.

It is well known that exercise boosts your wellbeing and instils a sense of discipline. All of which will reflect well in your revision. It's well worth devoting half an hour a day to some exercise, get your heart rate up, break a sweat, and get those endorphins flowing.

Sleep

It's no secret that when revising you need to keep well rested. Don't be tempted to stay up late revising as sleep actually plays an important part in consolidating long term memory. Instead aim for a minimum of 7 hours good sleep each night, in a dark room without any glow from electronic appliances. Install flux (https://justgetflux.com) on your laptop to prevent your computer from disrupting your circadian rhythm. Aim to go to bed the same time each night and no hitting snooze on the alarm clock in the morning!

Revision Timetable

Still struggling to get organised? Then try filling in the example revision timetable below, remember to factor in enough time for short breaks, and stick to it! Remember to schedule in several breaks throughout the day and actually use them to do something you enjoy e.g. TV, reading, YouTube etc.

	8AM	)AM	12P	2PM	4PM	6PM	8PM
IONDAY							
UESDAY							
IURSDAY							
'RIDAY							
.TURDAY							
'UNDAY							
XAMPLE DAY			School		Biology	Problem	hysics

ı have a much more accurate idea of the time you're spending on a question. In general, if you've spent 50 seconds on a section 1 question or >90 seconds on a section 2 questions – move on regardless of how close you think you are to solving it.

Getting the most out of Mock Papers

Mock exams can prove invaluable if tackled correctly. Not only do they encourage you to start revision earlier, they also allow you to **practice and perfect your revision technique**. They are often the best way of improving your knowledge base or reinforcing what you have learnt. Probably the best reason for attempting mock papers is to familiarise yourself with the exam conditions of the IMAT as they are particularly tough.

Start Revision Earlier

Thirty five percent of students agree that they procrastinate to a degree that is detrimental to their exam performance. This is partly explained by the fact that they often seem a long way in the future. In the scientific literature this is well recognised, Dr. Piers Steel, an expert on the field of motivation states that *'the further away an event is, the less impact it has on your decisions'*.

Mock exams are therefore a way of giving you a target to work towards and motivate you in the run up to the real thing – every time you do one treat it as the real deal! If you do well then it's a reassuring sign; if you do poorly then it will motivate you to work harder (and earlier!).

Practice and perfect revision techniques

In case you haven't realised already, revision is a skill all to itself, and can take some time to learn. For example, the most common revision techniques including **highlighting and/or re-reading are quite ineffective** ways of committing things to memory. Unless you are thinking critically about something you are much less likely to remember it or indeed understand it.

Mock exams, therefore allow you to test your revision strategies as you go along. Try spacing out your revision sessions so you have time to forget what you have learnt in-between. This may sound counterintuitive but the second time you remember it for longer. Try teaching another student what you have learnt, this forces you to structure the information in a logical way that may aid memory. Always try to question what you have learnt and appraise its validity. Not only does this aid memory but it is also a useful skill for IMAT section 3, Oxbridge interview, and beyond.

Improve your knowledge

The act of applying what you have learnt reinforces that piece of knowledge. A question may ask you to think about a relatively basic concept in a novel way (not cited in textbooks), and so deepen your understanding. Exams rarely test word for word what is in the syllabus, so when running through mock papers try to understand how the basic facts are applied and tested in the exam. As you go through the mocks or past papers take note of your performance and see if you consistently under-perform in specific areas, thus highlighting areas for future study.

Get familiar with exam conditions

Pressure can cause all sorts of trouble for even the most brilliant students. The IMAT is a particularly time pressured exam with high stakes – your future (without exaggerating) does depend on your result to a great extent. The real key to the IMAT is overcoming this pressure and remaining calm to allow you to think efficiently.

Mock exams are therefore an excellent opportunity to devise and perfect your own exam techniques to beat the pressure and meet the demands of the exam. **Don't treat mock exams like practice questions – it's imperative you do them under time conditions.**

'emember! It's better that you make all the mistakes you possibly can now in mock papers and then learn 'om them so as not to repeat them in the real exam.

Things to have done before using this book

Do the ground work

- Read in detail: the background, methods, and aims of the IMAT as well logistical considerations such as how to take the IMAT in practice. A good place to start is a IMAT textbook like *The Ultimate IMAT Guide* (flick to the back to get a free copy!) which covers all the groundwork but it's also worth looking through the official IMAT site (www.admissionstesting.org/IMAT).
- It is generally a good idea to start re-capping all your GCSE maths and science.
- Practice substituting formulas together to reach a more useful one expressing known variables e.g. P = IV and V= IR can be combined to give $P = V^2/R$ and $P = I^2R$. Remember that calculators are not permitted in the exam, so get comfortable doing more complex long addition, multiplication, division, and subtraction.
- Get comfortable rapidly converting between percentages, decimals, and fractions.
- Practice developing logical arguments and structuring essays with an obvious introduction, main body, and ending.
- These are all things which are easiest to do alongside your revision for exams before the summer break. Not only gaining a head start on your IMAT revision but also complimenting your year 12 studies well.
- Discuss scientific problems with others - propose experiments and state what you think the result would be. Be ready to defend your argument. This will rapidly build your scientific understanding for section 2 but also prepare you well for an oxbridge interview.
- Read through the IMAT syllabus before you start tackling whole papers. This is absolutely essential. It contains several stated formulae, constants, and facts that you are expected to apply - or may just be an answer in their own right. Familiarising yourself with the syllabus is also a quick way of teaching yourself the additional information other exam boards may learn which you do not. Sifting through the whole IMAT syllabus is a time-consuming process so we have done it for you. **Be sure to flick through the syllabus checklist** later on, which also doubles up as a great revision aid for the night before!

Ease in gently

With the ground work laid, there's still no point in adopting exam conditions straight away. Instead invest in a beginner's guide to the IMAT, which will not only describe in detail the background and theory of the exam, but take you through section by section what is expected. *The Ultimate IMAT Guide: 800 Practice Questions* is the most popular IMAT textbook – you can get a free copy by flicking to the back of this book.

When you are ready to move on to past papers, take your time and puzzle your way through all the questions. Really try to understand solutions. A past paper question won't be repeated in your real exam, so don't rote learn methods or facts. Instead, focus on applying prior knowledge to formulate your own approach.

If you're really struggling and have to take a sneak peek at the answers, then practice thinking of alternative solutions, or arguments for essays. It is unlikely that your answer will be more elegant or succinct than the model answer, but it is still a good task for encouraging creativity with your thinking. Get used to thinking outside the box!

Accelerate and Intensify

Start adopting exam conditions after you've done two past papers. Don't forget that **it's the time pressure that makes the IMAT hard** – if you had as long as you wanted to sit the exam you would probably get 100%. If you're struggling to find comprehensive answers to past papers then *IMAT Past Papers Worked Solutions* contains detailed explained answers to every IMAT past paper question and essay (flick to the back to get a free copy).

Doing all the past papers from 2009 – present is a good target for your revision. Note that the IMAT syllabus changed in 2009 so questions before this date may no longer be relevant. In any case, choose a paper and proceed with strict exam conditions. Take a short break and then mark your answers before reviewing your progress. For revision purposes, as you go along, keep track of those questions that you guess – these are equally as important to review as those you get wrong.

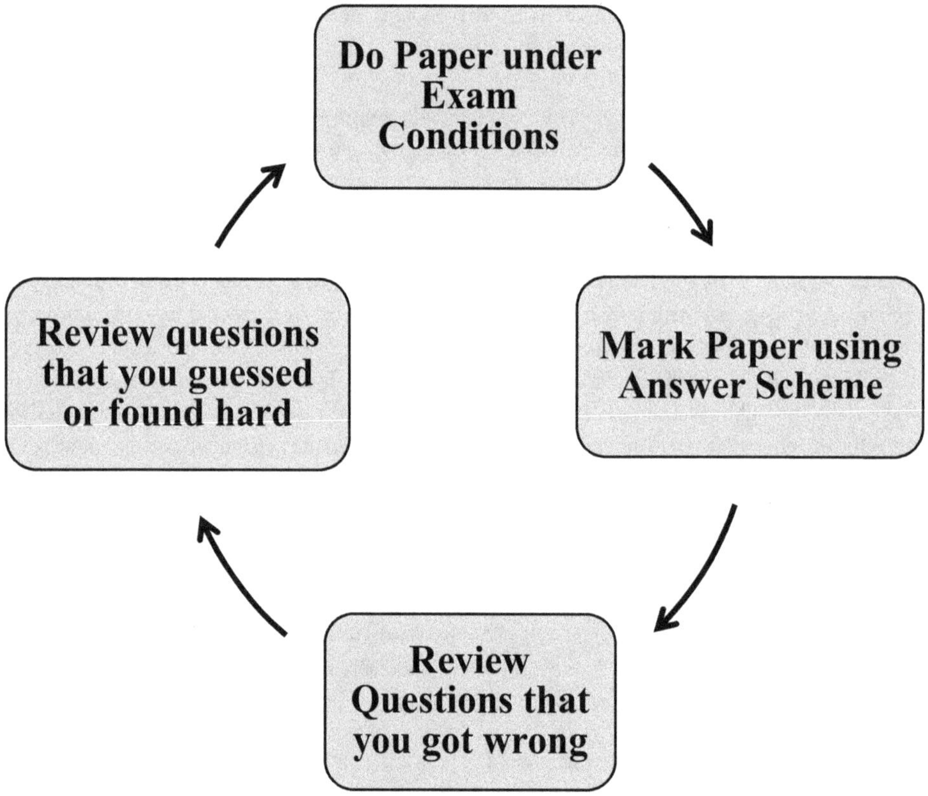

Once you've exhausted all the past papers, move on to tackling the unique mock papers in this book. In general, you should aim to complete one to two mock papers every night in the ten days preceding your exam.

Section 1: An Overview

	22 MCQs

This is the first section of the IMAT, comprising what most people describe as the classic IQ test style questions. Giving you one hour to answer 35 questions testing your ability to think critically, solve problems, and handle data. Breaking things down you realise that you are left with approximately 100 seconds per question. Remember though that this not only includes reasoning your answers, but also reading passages of text and/or analysing diagrams or graphs.

Not all the questions are of equal difficulty and so as you work through the past material it is certainly worth learning to recognise quickly which questions you need to skip to avoid getting bogged down. If it comes to it and you do not have enough time to go back to any skipped questions at the end, you always have a 20% chance of getting the answer correct with a guess!

Critical thinking questions

These types of question will generally present you with a passage of text or a methodology for an experiment and ask you to do one of three things: identify a conclusion, identify and assumption or flaw, or give an argument to either strengthen or weaken the statement.

The ability to filter through irrelevant material is essential with these questions as well as a solid grasp of the English language. Remember to only use the information given to you in your reasoning and never be too general with your conclusions – seek direct evidence in the information given. Critical thinking questions are definitely an example of when it is **best to read the question first**!

Problem solving questions

The problems in section 1 are often very wordy and complex, therefore it is often useful to turn the prose of the question into a series of equations. For example, being able to turn the sentence "Megan is half as tall as Elin" into "2M = E" should become second nature to you. Trial and error is not a method you should adopt for any questions in section 1 as it is far too time consuming.

As you are working through the preparation material try to get used to recognising which questions can be aided by drawing a quick diagram. This could apply to questions asking about timetables, orders, sequences, or spatial relationships. Remember it doesn't have to be pretty, merely help you organise your thoughts!

Data handling questions

These questions will undoubtedly require you to work with numbers, often calculating percentages or frequencies. Again, reading the question first can help you save time here, directing your attention to the relevant information in the passage. When analysing tables or graphs always check the following:

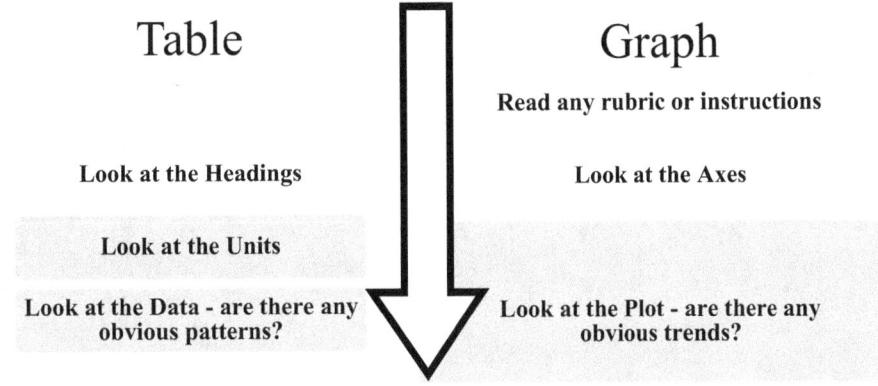

Table	Graph
	Read any rubric or instructions
Look at the Headings	**Look at the Axes**
Look at the Units	
Look at the Data - are there any obvious patterns?	**Look at the Plot - are there any obvious trends?**

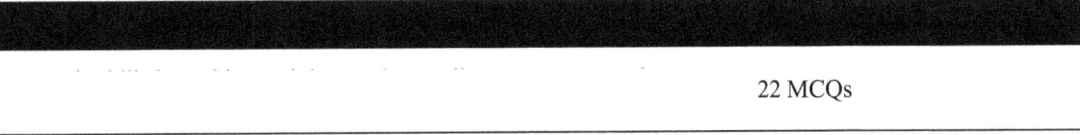

Sections 2, 3 & 4: An Overview

What will you be tested on?	No. of Questions	Duration
Ability to recall, understand and apply scientific knowledge and principles of biology, chemistry, physics, and maths. Usually the sections that students find the hardest.	38 MCQs	65 Minutes

If you're short of time, then these sections are where to focus. Undoubtedly the most time pressured section of the IMAT (requiring you to answer a question every 100 seconds) but also the section where candidates improve the fastest. These sections draw on your knowledge of biology, chemistry, physics, and maths.

Biology

Generally, the biology questions require the least amount of time and are often where you can rely on making up lost time from harder questions. Most of biology questions rely on you being able to recall facts rather than interpret data or solve equations, so some good old-fashioned text book revision will prepare you well for these questions.

Chemistry

If you're taking the IMAT you will undoubtedly be studying chemistry at A-level as it is a requirement of all medical schools. Conceptually therefore, you should be in the clear, however, balancing complex equations or processing lengthy calculations can be time consuming.

Practicing with mock papers is essentially in combating this – really focus on extracting what the question is asking for as quickly as possible. In addition to the equations on the subsequent pages you must be comfortable with converting between litres, dm^3, cm^3, and mm^3 as well as using Avogadro's constant in calculations.

Physics

Physics is by far the most common subject that students drop moving on to AS-level, meaning these questions are the most poorly answered. There is a large variation in physics specifications between GCSE exam boards, so **before you do anything else read through the IMAT syllabus and commit all the stated equations and constants to memory** (helpfully highlighted in bold type on the revision checklist).

Physics questions will almost always require a two-step solution, normally forcing you to combine and re-arrange equations. All answers must be given in SI units which actually benefits you, by looking at the units you can often derive the equation – for example speed in m/s is calculated as distance(m) / time(s). It is also worth becoming fluent with the terminology for orders of magnitude in measurements (see right).

Factor	Text	Symbol
10^{12}	Tera	T
10^{9}	Giga	G
10^{6}	Mega	M
10^{3}	Kilo	k
10^{2}	Hecto	h
10^{-1}	Deci	d
10^{-2}	Centi	c
10^{-3}	Milli	m
10^{-6}	Micro	μ
10^{-9}	Nano	n
10^{-12}	Pico	p

Maths

Maths is the single most important component of section 2, a question topic in its own right but also applied in chemistry, physics, and section 1. Just remember to limit yourself to GCSE knowledge in the maths questions and don't overcomplicate things. As a bare minimum for preparation you should practice applying the quadratic formula, completing the square, and finding the difference between 2 squares.

How to use this Book

If you have done everything this book has described so far then you should be well equipped to meet the demands of the IMAT, and therefore **the mock papers in the rest of this book should ONLY be completed under exam conditions**.

This means:

- Absolute silence – no TV or music
- Absolute focus – no distractions such as eating your dinner
- Strict time constraints – no pausing half way through
- No checking the answers as you go
- Give yourself a maximum of three minutes between sections – keep the pressure up
- Complete the entire paper before marking
- Mark harshly

In practice this means setting aside two hours in an evening to find a quiet spot without interruptions and tackle the paper. Completing one mock paper every evening in the week running up to the exam would be an ideal target.

- Tackle the paper as you would in the exam.
- Return to mark your answers, but mark harshly if there's any ambiguity.
- Highlight any areas of concern.
- If warranted read up on the areas you felt you underperformed to reinforce your knowledge.
- If you inadvertently learnt anything new by muddling through a question, go and tell somebody about it to reinforce what you've discovered.

Finally relax… the IMAT is an exhausting exam, concentrating so hard continually for two hours will take its toll. So, being able to relax and switch off is essential to keep yourself sharp for exam day! Make sure you reward yourself after you finish marking your exam.

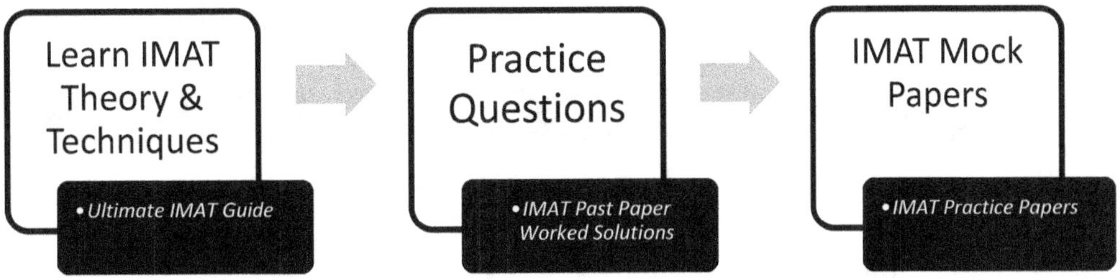

Scoring Tables

Use these to keep a record of your scores from past papers – you can then easily see which paper you should attempt next (always the one with the lowest score).

SECTION 1	1st Attempt	2nd Attempt	3rd Attempt
2011			
2012			
2013			
2014			
2015			
2016			
2017			
2018			

SECTION 2	1st Attempt	2nd Attempt	3rd Attempt
2011			
2012			
2013			
2014			
2015			
2016			
2017			
2018			

SECTION 3	1st Attempt	2nd Attempt	3rd Attempt
2011			
2012			
2013			
2014			
2015			
2016			
2017			
2018			

SECTION 4	1st Attempt	2nd Attempt	3rd Attempt
2011			
2012			
2013			
2014			
2015			
2016			
2017			
2018			

And the same again here but with our mocks instead.

SECTION 1	1st Attempt	2nd Attempt	3rd Attempt
Mock A			
Mock B			
Mock C			
Mock D			
Mock E			
Mock F			
Mock G			
Mock H			

SECTION 2	1st Attempt	2nd Attempt	3rd Attempt
Mock A			
Mock B			
Mock C			
Mock D			
Mock E			
Mock F			
Mock G			
Mock H			

SECTION 3	1st Attempt	2nd Attempt	3rd Attempt
Mock A			
Mock B			
Mock C			
Mock D			
Mock E			
Mock F			
Mock G			
Mock H			

SECTION 4	1st Attempt	2nd Attempt	3rd Attempt
Mock A			
Mock B			
Mock C			
Mock D			
Mock E			
Mock F			
Mock G			
Mock H			

MOCK PAPER A

Section 1

Question 1:
A square sheet of paper is 20cms long. How many times must it be folded in half before it covers an area of 12.5cm^2?

A) 3 B) 4 C) 5 D) 6 E) 7

Question 2:
Mountain climbing is viewed by some as an extreme sport, while for others it is simply an exhilarating pastime that offers the ultimate challenge of strength, endurance, and sacrifice. It can be highly dangerous, even fatal, especially when the climber is out of his or her depth, or simply gets overwhelmed by weather, terrain, ice, or other dangers of the mountain. Inexperience, poor planning, and inadequate equipment can all contribute to injury or death, so knowing what to do right matters.

Despite all the negatives, when done right, mountain climbing is an exciting, exhilarating, and rewarding experience. This article is an overview beginner's guide and outlines the initial basics to learn. Each step is deserving of an article in its own right, and entire tomes have been written on climbing mountains, so you're advised to spend a good deal of your beginner's learning immersed in reading widely. This basic overview will give you an idea of what is involved in a climb.

Which statement best summarises this paragraph?
A) Mountain climbing is an extreme sport fraught with dangers.
B) Without extensive experience embarking on a mountain climb is fatal.
C) A comprehensive literature search is the key to enjoying mountain climbing.
D) Mountain climbing is difficult and is a skill that matures with age if pursued.
E) The terrain is the biggest unknown when climbing a mountain and therefore presents the biggest danger.

Question 3:
50% of an isolated population contract a new strain of resistant Malaria. Only 20% are symptomatic of which 10% are female. What percentage of the total population do symptomatic males represent?

A) 1% B) 9% C) 10% D) 80%

Question 4:
John is a UK citizen yet is looking to buy a holiday home in the South of France. He is purchasing his new home through an agency. Unlike a normal estate agent, they offer monthly discount sales of up to 30%. As a French company, the agency sells in Euros. John decides to hold off on his purchase until the sale in the interest of saving money. What is the major assumption made in doing this?

A) The house he likes will not be bought in the meantime.
B) The agency will not be declared bankrupt.
C) The value of the pound will fall more than 30%.
D) The value of the pound will fall less than 30%.
E) The value of the euro may increase by up to 35% in the coming weeks.

Question 5:
In childcare professions, by law, there must be an adult to child ratio of no more than 1:4. Child minders are hired on a salary of £8.50 an hour. What is the maximum number of children that can be continually supervised for a period of 24 hours on a budget of £1,000?
A) 1 B) 8 C) 12 D) 16 E) 468

Question 6:
A table of admission prices for the local cinema is shown below:

	Peak	Off-peak
Adult	£11	£9.50
Child	£7	£5.50
Concession	£7	£5.50
Student	£5	£5

How much would a group of 3 adults, 5 children, a concession and 4 students save by visiting at an off-peak time rather than a peak time?

A) £11.50 B) £13.50 C) £15.50 D) £17.50 E) £18.50

Question 7:
All musicians play instruments. All oboe players are musicians. Oboes and pianos are instruments. Karen is a musician. Which statement is true?

A) Karen plays two instruments.
B) All musicians are oboe players.
C) All instruments are pianos or oboes.
D) Karen is an oboe player.
E) None of the above.

Question 8:
Flow mediated dilatation is a method used to assess vascular function within the body. It essentially adopts the use of an ultrasound scan to measure the percentage increase in the width of an artery before and after occlusion with a blood pressure cuff. Ultrasound scans are taken by one sonographer, and the average lumen diameter is then measured by an analyst. What is a potential flaw in the methodology of this technique?

A) Results will not be comparable within an individual if different arteries start at different diameters.
B) Results will not be comparable between individuals if they have different baseline arterial diameters.
C) Ultrasound is an outdated technique with no use in modern medicine.
D) This methodology is subject to human error.
E) This methodology is not repeatable.

Question 9:
If it takes 20 minutes to board an aeroplane, 15 minutes to disembark and the flight lasts two and a half hours. In the event of a delay it is not uncommon to add 20 minutes to the flight time. Megan is catching the flight in question as she needs to attend a meeting at 5pm. The location of the meeting is 15 minutes from the airport without traffic; 25 minutes with. Which of the following statements is valid considering this information?

A) If Megan wants to be on time for her meeting, given all possibilities described, the latest she can begin boarding at the departure airport is 1.30pm.
B) If Megan starts boarding at 1.40pm she will certainly be late.
C) If Megan aims to start boarding at 1.10pm she will arrive in time whether the plane is delayed or not.
D) If Megan wishes to be on time she doesn't have to worry about the plane being delayed as she can make up the time during the transport time from the arrival airport to the meeting.

Question 10:
A cask of whiskey holds a total volume of 500L. Every two and a half minutes half of the total volume is collected and discarded. How many minutes will it take for the entire cask to be emptied?

A) 80 B) 160 C) 200 D) 240 E) ∞

Question 11:

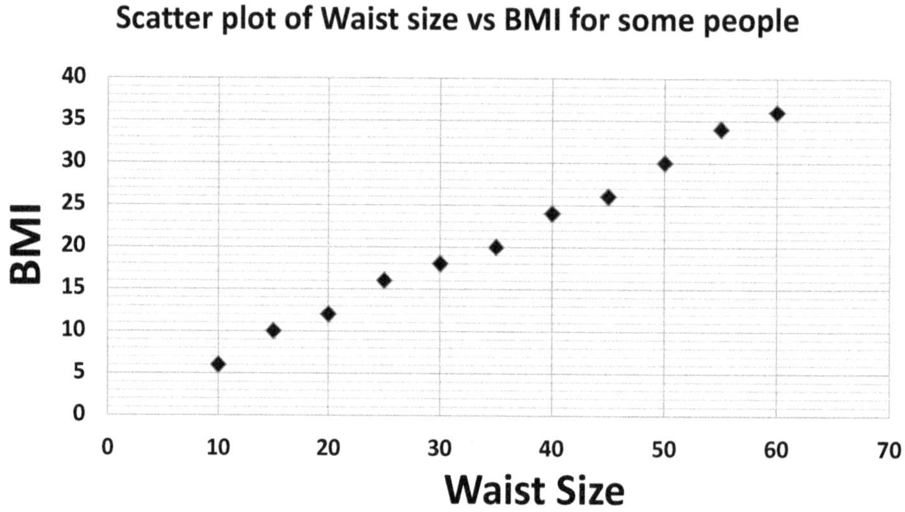

What can be concluded from the graph above?

A) Having a larger waist size causes an increase in BMI.
B) Having a larger BMI causes an increase in waist size.
C) Waist size is reciprocal to BMI.
D) No conclusions can be drawn from this graph.
E) None of the above are correct.

Question 12:
B is right of A. C is left of B. D is in front of C. E is in front of B. Where is D in relation to E?

A) D is behind E.
B) E is behind D.
C) D is to the right of E.
D) D is to the left of E.
E) E is to the left of D.

Question 13:
Car A has a fuel tank capacity of 30 gallons and achieves 40mpg. Car B on the other hand has a fuel tank capacity of 50 gallons but only achieves 30mpg. Both cars drive until they run out of fuel. If car A starts with a full tank of petrol and travels 200 miles further than car B, how full was car B's fuel tank?

A) 1/5 B) 1/4 C) 1/3 D) 1/2 E) 2/3

Question 14:
The keypad to a safe comprises the digits 1 - 9. The code itself can be of indeterminate length. The code is therefore set by choosing a reference number so that when a code is entered the average of all the numbers entered must equal the chosen reference number.

Which of the following is true?

A) If the reference number was set greater than 9, the safe would be locked forever.
B) This safe is extremely insecure as if random digits were pressed for long enough it would average out at the correct reference number.
C) More than one number is always required to achieve the reference number.
D) All of the above are true.
E) None of the above are true.

Question 15:
The use of antibiotics is one of the major paradoxes in modern medicine. Antibiotics themselves provide a selection pressure to drive the evolution of antibiotic resistant strains of bacteria. This is largely due to the rapid growth rate of bacterial colonies and asexual cell division. As such a widespread initiative is in place to limit the prescription of antibiotics.
Which of the following is a fair assumption?

A) Antibiotic resistance is impossible to avoid as it is driven by evolution.
B) If bacteria reproduced at a slower rate antibiotic resistance would not be such an issue.
C) Medicine always creates more problems than it solves.
D) In the past antibiotics were used frivolously.
E) All of the above could be possible.

<u>The information below relates to questions 16 – 20:</u>

The Spaghetti Bolognese recipe below serves 10 people and each portion contains 300 kcal.

- 1kg mince
- 220g pancetta, diced
- 30g crushed garlic
- 1kg tinned tomatoes
- 300g diced onions
- 300g sliced mushrooms
- 200g grated cheese

Question 16:
What quantity of cheese is required to prepare a meal for 350 people?

A) 0.7kg B) 7kg C) 70kg D) 700kg E) 7000kg

Question 17:
If 12 portions represent 120% of an individual's recommended calorific intake, what is that individuals recommended calorific intake?

A) 2600kcal B) 2800kcal C) 3000kcal D) 3200kcal E) 3400kcal

Question 18:
The recommended ratio of pasta to Bolognese is 4:1. If cooking for 30 people how much pasta should be used?

A) 30.3kg B) 36.6kg C) 42.9kg D) 49.2kg E) 55.5kg

Question 19:
What is the ratio of onions to the rest of the ingredients if garlic and pancetta are ignored?

F) 1/2.05 G) 1/3.9 H) 1/6.7 I) 1/9.3 J) 1/10

Question 20:
It takes 4 minutes to prepare the ingredients per portion, and a further 8 minutes per portion to cook. Simon has ample preparation space but is limited to cooking 8 portions at a time. What is the shortest period of time it would take him to turn all the ingredients into a meal for 25 people, assuming he didn't start cooking until all the ingredients were prepared?

A) 3 hours
B) 3 hours 40
C) 4 hours
D) 4 hours 40
E) 5 hours

Question 21:
Who wrote *Don Quixote*?

A) William Shakespeare
B) Miguel de Cervantes
C) Jorge Luis Borges
D) Lope de Vega
E) Victor Hugo

Question 22:
Where did the Orange Revolution take place in 2004?

A) Georgia
B) Czechoslovakia
C) Lebanon
D) Ukraine
E) Philippines

END OF SECTION

Section 2

Question 23:

Which of the following cannot be classified as an organ?

1. Blood
2. Bone
3. Larynx
4. Pituitary Gland
5. Prostate
6. Skeletal Muscle
7. Skin

A) 1 and 6 B) 2 and 3 C) 5 and 7 D) 1 and 5 E) 1,4, 5 and 6

Question 24:

An increase in aerobic respiratory rate could be associated with which of the following physiological changes?

1. A larger percentage of water vapour in expired air
2. Increased expired CO_2
3. Increased inspired O_2
4. Perspiration
5. Vasodilatation

A) 3 only
B) 1 and 2 only
C) 1, 2 and 3 only
D) 2, 3 and 5
E) All of the above

Question 25:

The nephron is to the kidney, as the ________ is to striated muscle:

A) Actin filament
B) Artery
C) Myofibril
D) Sarcomere
E) Vein

Question 26:

A diabetic patient's glucagon and insulin levels are measured over 4 hours. During this time the patient is given two large boluses of glucose. A graphical representation of this is shown below.

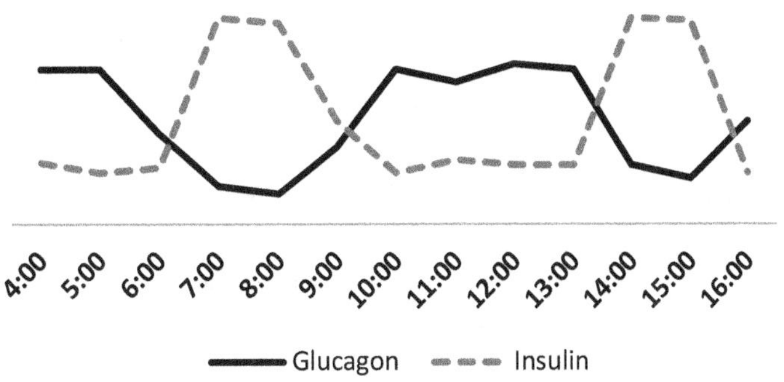

At which times would you expect the patients' blood glucose to be greatest?

A) 05:00 and 12:00
B) 07:00 and 14.00
C) 08:00 and 15:00
D) 10:00 and 13:00
E) 06:00, 10:00 and 16:00

Question 27:

In addition to the A, B or O classification, blood groups can also be distinguished by the presence of Rhesus antigen (Rh). Care must be taken in blood transfusion as once blood types are mixed a Rh -ve individual will mount an immune response against Rh +ve blood. This is particular well exemplified in haemolytic disease of the newborn – where a Rh-ve mother carries a Rh+ve foetus.

Applying what is written here and your knowledge of the human immune system, explain why the mother's first child would be relatively safe and unaffected, yet further offspring would be at high risk.

A) The first pregnancy is always such a shock to the body it compromises the immune system.
B) Antibodies take longer than 9 months to produce and mature to an active state.
C) First born children are immunologically privileged.
D) There is a high risk of haemorrhage to both mother and child during birth.
E) Plasma T cells require time to multiply to lethal levels.

Question 28:

At present a large effort is being made to produce tailored patient care. One of the ultimate goals of this is to be able to grow personal, genetically identical organs for those with end stage organ failure. This process will first require the harbouring of what cell type?

A) Cells from the organ that is failing
B) Haematopoietic stem cells
C) Embryonic stem cells
D) Adult stem cells
E) All of the above

Question 29:

In relation to the human genome, which of the following are correct?

1. The DNA genome is coded by 4 different bases.
2. The sugar backbone of the DNA strand is formed of glucose.
3. DNA is found in the nucleus of bacteria.

A) 1 only
B) 2 only
C) 3 only
D) 1 and 2
E) 1 and 3
F) 2 and 3
G) 1, 2 and 3

Question 30:

Animal cells contain organelles that take part in vital processes. Which of the following is true?

1. The majority of energy production by animal cells occurs in the mitochondria.
2. The cell wall protects the animal cell membrane from outside pressure differences.
3. The endoplasmic reticulum plays a role in protein synthesis.

A) 1 only
B) 2 only
C) 3 only
D) 1 and 2
E) 2 and 3
F) 1 and 3
G) 1, 2 and 3

Question 31:
With regards to animal mitochondria, which of the following is correct?

A) Mitochondria are not necessary for aerobic respiration.
B) Mitochondria are the sole cause of sperm cell movement.
C) The majority of DNA replication happens inside mitochondria.
D) Mitochondria are more abundant in fat cells than in skeletal muscle.
E) The majority of protein synthesis occurs in mitochondria.
F) Mitochondria are enveloped by a double membrane.

Question 32:
In relation to bacteria, which of the following is **FALSE**?

A) Bacteria always lead to disease.
B) Bacteria contain plasmid DNA.
C) Bacteria do not contain mitochondria.
D) Bacteria have a cell wall and a plasma membrane.
E) Some bacteria are susceptible to antibiotics.

Question 33:
In relation to bacterial replication, which of the following is correct?

A) Bacteria undergo sexual reproduction.
B) Bacteria have a nucleus.
C) Bacteria carry genetic information on circular plasmids.
D) Bacterial genomes are formed of RNA instead of DNA.
E) Bacteria require gametes to replicate.

Question 34:
Which of the following are correct regarding active transport?

A) ATP is necessary and sufficient for active transport.
B) ATP is not necessary but sufficient for active transport.
C) The relative concentrations of the material being transported have little impact on the rate of active transport.
D) Transport proteins are necessary and sufficient for active transport.
E) Active transport relies on transport proteins that are powered by an electrochemical gradient.

Question 35:
Concerning mammalian reproduction, which of the following is **FALSE**?

A) Fertilisation involves the fusion of two gametes.
B) Reproduction is sexual and the offspring display genetic variation.
C) Reproduction relies upon the exchange of genetic material.
D) Mammalian gametes are diploid cells produced via meiosis.
E) Embryonic growth requires carefully controlled mitosis.

Question 36:
Which of the following apply to Mendelian inheritance?

1. It only applies to plants.
2. It treats different traits as either dominant or recessive.
3. Heterozygotes have a 25% chance of expressing a recessive trait.

A) 1 only
B) 2 only
C) 3 only
D) 1 and 2
E) 1 and 3
F) 2 and 3
G) All of the above

Question 37:
Which of the following statements are correct?

A) Hormones are secreted into the blood stream and act over long distances at specific target organs.
B) Hormones are substances that almost always cause muscles to contract.
C) Hormones have no impact on the nervous or enteric systems.
D) Hormones are always derived from food and never synthesised.
E) Hormones act rapidly to restore homeostasis.

Question 38:
With regard to neuronal signalling in the body, which of the following are true?

1. Neuronal transmission can be caused by both electrical and chemical stimulation.
2. Synapses ultimately result in the production of an electrical current for signal transduction.
3. All synapses in humans are electrical and unidirectional.

A) 1 only
B) 2 only
C) 3 only
D) 1 and 2
E) 1 and 3
F) 2 and 3
G) 1, 2 and 3

Question 39:
What is the **primary** reason that pH is controlled so tightly in humans?

A) To allow rapid protein synthesis.
B) To allow for effective digestion throughout the GI tract.
C) To ensure ions can function properly in neural signalling.
D) To prevent changes in electrical charge in polypeptide chains.
E) To prevent changes in core body temperature.

Question 40:
Which of the following statements are correct regarding bacterial cell walls?

1. It confers bacteria protection against external environmental stimuli.
2. It is an evolutionary remnant and now has little functional significance in most bacteria.
3. It is made up primarily of glucose in bacteria.

A) Only 1
B) Only 2
C) Only 3
D) 1 and 2
E) 2 and 3
F) 1 and 3
G) 1, 2 and 3

END OF SECTION

Section 3

Question 41:
The pH of a solution has the greatest effect on which type of interaction?

A) Van der Waals
B) Induced dipole
C) Ionic bonding
D) Metallic interaction
E) Hydrogen bonding

Question 42:
When comparing different isotopes of the same element, which of the following may change?

1. Atomic number
2. Mass number
3. Number of electrons
4. Chemical reactivity

A) 1 only
B) 1 and 2 only
C) 3 only
D) 2 and 3 only
E) All of the above

Question 43:
From which of the following elemental groups are you most likely to find a catalyst?

A) Alkali Metals
B) d-block elements
C) Alkaline Earth Metals
D) Noble Gases
E) Halogens

Question 44:
1.338kg of francium are mixed in a reaction vessel with an excess of distilled water. What volume will the hydrogen produced occupy at room temperature and pressure?

A) $20.4dm^3$
B) $36dm^3$
C) $40.8dm^3$
D) $60.12dm^3$
E) $72dm^3$

Question 45:
The composition of a compound is Carbon 30%, Hydrogen 40%, Fluorine 20%, and Chlorine 10%. What is the empirical formula of this compound?

A) CH_2FCl
B) $C_3H_2F_2Cl$
C) C_3H_4FCl
D) $C_3H_4F_2Cl$
E) $C_4H_4F_2Cl$

Question 46:
What is the actual molecular formula of the compound in question 13 if the M_r is 340.5?

A) $C_3H_4F_2Cl$
B) $C_6H_8F_4Cl_2$
C) $C_9H_{12}F_6Cl_3$
D) $C_{12}H_{16}F_8Cl_4$
E) $C_{15}H_{20}F_{10}Cl_5$

Question 47:
1.2×10^{10} kg of sugar is dissolved in 4×10^{12}L of distilled water. What is the concentration?

A) 3×10^{-2} g/dL
B) 3×10^{-1} g/dL
C) 3×10^{1} g/dL
D) 3×10^{2} g/dL
E) 3×10^{3} g/dL

Question 48:
Which of the following is not essential for the progression of an exothermic chemical reaction?

A) Presence of a catalyst
B) Increase in entropy
C) Achieving activation energy
D) Attaining an electron configuration more closely resembling that of a noble gas
E) None of the above

Question 49:
What is a common use of cationic surfactants?

A) Shampoo
B) Lubricant
C) Cosmetics
D) Detergents
E) All of the above

Question 50:
Which of the following most accurately defines an isotope?

A) An isotope is an atom of an element that has the same number of protons in the nucleus but a different number of neutrons orbiting the nucleus.
B) An isotope is an atom of an element that has the same number of neutrons in the nucleus but a different number of protons orbiting the nucleus.
C) An isotope is any atom of an element that can be split to produce nuclear energy.
D) An isotope is an atom of an element that has the same number of protons in the nucleus but a different number of neutrons in the nucleus.
E) An isotope is an atom of an element that has the same number of protons in the nucleus but a different number of electrons orbiting it.

Question 51:
Which of the following is an example of a displacement reaction?

1. $Fe + SnSO4 \rightarrow FeSO_4 + Sn$
2. $Cl_2 + 2KBr \rightarrow Br_2 + 2KCl$
3. $H_2SO_4 + Mg \rightarrow MgSO_4 + H_2$
4. $NaHCO_3 + HCl \rightarrow NaCl + CO_2 + H_2O$

A) 1 only
B) 1 and 2 only
C) 2 and 3 only
D) 3 and 4 only
E) 1, 2 and 3 only
F) 1,2, 3 and 4

Question 52:
What values of **a**, **b** and **c** are needed to balance the equation below?

$\mathbf{a}Ca(OH)_2 + \mathbf{b}H_3PO_4 \rightarrow Ca_3(PO_4)_2 + \mathbf{c}H_2O$

A) a = 3 b = 2 c = 6
B) a = 2 b = 2 c = 4
C) a = 3 b = 2 c = 1
D) a = 1 b = 2 c = 3
E) a = 4 b = 2 c = 6
F) a = 3 b = 2 c = 4

END OF SECTION

Section 4

Question 53:
A crocodile's tail weighs 30kg. Its head weighs as much as the tail and one half of the body and legs. The body and legs together weigh as much as the tail and head combined.

What is the total weight of the crocodile?

A) 220kg B) 240kg C) 260kg D) 280kg E) 300kg

Question 54:
A body is travelling at x ms^{-1} with y J of kinetic energy. After a period of retardation the kinetic energy of the body is $1/16y$. Assuming that the mass of the body has remained constant what is its new velocity?

A) $1/196x$ B) $1/16x$ C) $1/8x$ D) $1/4x$ E) $4x$

Question 55:
Which of the following is a unit equivalent to the Volt?

A) A.Ω^{-1} B) J.C^{-1} C) W.s^{-1} D) C.s E) W.C.Ω

Question 56:
Complete the sentence below:
A voltmeter is connected in _____ and therefore has _____ resistance; whereas an ammeter is connected in _____ and has _____ resistance.

A) Parallel, zero, parallel, infinite
B) Parallel, zero, series, infinite
C) Parallel, infinite, series, zero
D) Series, zero, parallel, infinite
E) Series, infinite, parallel, zero

Question 57:
A body "A" of mass 12kg travelling at 15m/s undergoes inelastic collision with a fixed, stationary object "B" of mass 20kg over a period of 0.5 seconds. After the collision body A has a new velocity of 3m/s. What force must have been dissipated during the collision?

A) 288N B) 298N C) 308N D) 318N E) 328N

Question 58:
What process is illustrated here: ${}^{14}_{6}C \rightarrow {}^{14}_{7}N + x$

A) Thermal decomposition
B) Alpha decay
C) Beta decay
D) Gamma decay

Question 59:
A radio dish is broadcasting messages into deep space on a 20 Hz radio frequency of wavelength 3km. With every hour how much further does the signal travel into deep space?

A) 200,000 km
B) 216,000 km
C) 232,000 km
D) 248,000 km
E) 264,000 km

Question 60:

A formula: $\sqrt[3]{\frac{z(x+y)(l+m-n)}{3}}$ is given. Would you expect this formula to calculate:

A) A length
B) An area
C) A volume
D) A volume of rotation
E) A geometric average

END OF PAPER

MOCK PAPER B

Section 1

Question 1:
"If vaccinations are now compulsory because society has decided that they should be forced, then society should pay for them." Which of the following statements would weaken the argument?

A) Many people disagree that vaccinations should be compulsory.
B) The cost of vaccinations is too high to be funded locally.
C) Vaccinations are supported by many local communities and GPs.
D) Healthcare workers do not want vaccinations.
E) None of the above

Question 2:
Josh is painting the outside walls of his house. The paint he has chosen is sold only in 10L tins. Each tin costs £4.99. Assuming a litre of paint covers an area of $5m^2$, and the total surface area of Josh's outside walls is $1050m^2$; what is the total cost of the paint required if Josh wants to apply 3 coats?

A) £104.79 B) £209.58 C) £314.37 D) £419.16 E) £523.95

Question 3:
The stars of the night sky have remained unchanged for many hundreds of years, which allows sailors to navigate using the North Star still to this day. However, this only applies within the northern hemisphere as the populations of the southern hemisphere are subject to an alternative night sky.

An asterism can be used to locate the North Star, it comes by many names including the plough, the saucepan, and the big dipper. Whilst the North Star's position remains fixed in the sky (allowing it to point north reliably always) the rest of the stars traverse around the North Star in a singular motion. In a very long time, the North Star will one day move from its location due to the movement of the Earth.

Which of the following is **NOT** an assumption made in this argument?

A) The Earth is rotating on its axis.
B) Sailors still have need to navigate using the stars.
C) An analogous southern star is used to navigate in the Southern hemisphere.
D) The plough is not the only method of locating the North Star.
E) None of the above.

Question 4:
John wishes to deposit a cheque. The bank's opening times are 9am until 5pm Monday to Friday, 10am until 4pm on Saturdays, and the bank is closed on Sundays. It takes on average 42 bank hours for the money from a cheque to become available.

If John needs the money by 8pm Tuesday, what is the latest he can cash the cheque?

A) 5pm the Saturday before
B) 5pm the Friday before
C) 1pm the Thursday before
D) 1pm the Wednesday before
E) 9am the Tuesday before

Question 5:

How many different diamonds are there in the image shown to the right?

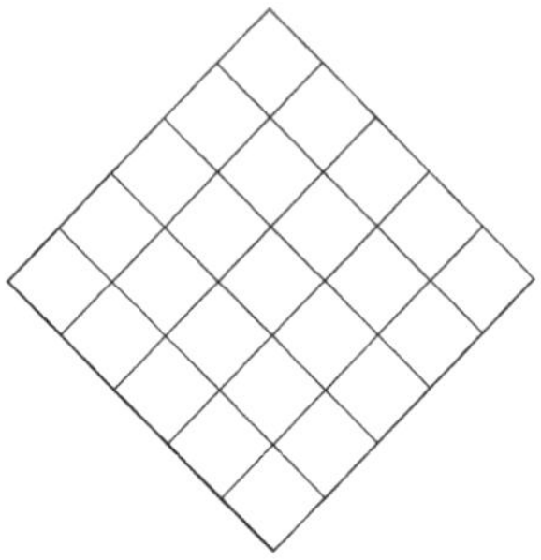

A) 25
B) 32
C) 48
D) 58
E) 63

Question 6:

In 4 years time I will be one third the age that my brother will be next year. In 20 years time he will be double my age. How old am I?

A) 4 B) 9 C) 15 D) 17 E) 23

Question 7:

Aneurysmal disease has been proven to induce systemic inflammatory effects, reaching far beyond the site of the aneurysm. The inflammatory mediator responsible for these processes remains unknown, however the effects of systemic inflammation have been well categorised and observed experimentally in pig models.

This inflammation induces an aberration of endothelial function within the inner most layer of blood vessel walls. The endothelium not only represents the lining of blood vessels but also acts as a transducer converting the haemodynamic forces of blood into a biological response. An example of this is the NO pathway, which uses the shear stress induced by increased blood flow to drive the formation of NO. NO diffuses from the endothelium into the smooth muscle surrounding blood vessels to promote vasodilatation and therefore acts to reduce blood flow. Failure of this process induces high risk of vascular damage and therefore cardiovascular diseases such as thrombosis and atherosclerosis.

What is a valid implication from the text above?

A) Aneurysmal disease does not affect the NO pathway.
B) Aneurysms directly increase the likelihood of cardiovascular disease.
C) Aneurysms are the opposite of transducers.
D) Observations of this kind should be made in humans to see if the results can be replicated.
E) Aneurysms induce high blood flow.

Question 8:

A traffic surveyor is stood at a T-junction between a main road and a side street. He is only interested in traffic leaving the side street. He logs the class of vehicle, the colour and the direction of travel once on the main road. During an 8-hour period he observes a total of 346 vehicles including bikes. Of which 200 were travelling west whilst the rest travelled east. The overwhelming majority of vehicles seen were cars at 90%, with bikes, vans and articulated lorries together comprising the remaining 10%. Red was the most common colour observed whilst green was the least. Black and white vehicles were seen in equal quantities.

Which of the following is an accurate inference based on this survey?

A) Global sales are highest for those vehicles which are coloured red.
B) Cars are the most popular vehicle on all roads.
C) Green vehicle sales are down in the area that the surveyor was based.
D) The daily average rate of traffic out of a T junction in Britain is 346 vehicles over 8 hours.
E) To the east of the junction is a dead end.

Question 9:
William, Xavier, and Yolanda race in a 100m race. All of them run at a constant speed during the race. William beats Xavier by 20m. Xavier beats Yolanda by 20m. How many metres does William beat Yolanda?

A) 30m B) 36m C) 40m D) 60m E) 64m

Question 10:
A television is delivered in a box that has volume 60% larger than that of the television. The television is 150cm x 100cm x 10m. How much surplus volume is there?

A) $0.09m^2$ B) $0.9\ m^2$ C) $9\ m^2$ D) $90\ m^2$ E) $900\ m^2$

Question 11:
Matthew and David are deciding where they would like to go camping Friday to Sunday. Upon completing their research, they discover the following:

- Whitmore Bay charges £5.50 a night and does not require a booking. The site provides showers, washing up facilities and easy access to a beach
- Port Eynon charges £5 a night and a booking is compulsory. However, the site does not provide showers but does have 240V sockets free of charge
- Jackson Bay charges £7 a night and is billed as a luxury site with compulsory booking, private showers, toilets, mobile phone charging facilities and kitchens.

David presents the following suggestion:
As Port Eynon is the farthest distance to travel the benefit of its cheap nightly rate is negated by the cost of petrol. Instead he recommends they visit Jackson Bay as it is the shortest distance to travel and will therefore be the cheapest.

Which of the following best illustrates a flaw in this argument?

A) Whitmore bay may be only a few miles further which means the total cost would be less than visiting Jackson Bay.
B) With kitchen facilities available they will be tempted to buy more food increasing the cost.
C) The campsite may be fully booked.
D) There may be a booking fee driving the cost up above that of the other campsites.
E) All of the above.

Question 12:
The manufacture of any new pharmaceutical is not permitted without scrupulous testing and analysis. This has led to the widespread, and controversial use of animal models in science. Whilst it is possible to test cyto-toxicity on simple cell cultures, to truly predict the effect of a drug within a physiological system it must be trialled in a whole organism. With animals cheap to maintain, readily available, rapidly reproducing and not subject to the same strict ethical laws they have become an invaluable component of modern scientific practice.

Which of the following best illustrates the main conclusion of this argument?

A) New pharmaceuticals cannot be approved without animal experimentation.
B) Cell culture experiments are unhelpful.
C) Modern medicine would not have achieved its current standard without animal experimentation.
D) Logistically animals are easier to keep than humans for mandatory experiments.
E) All of the above.

The information below relates to questions 13 – 17:

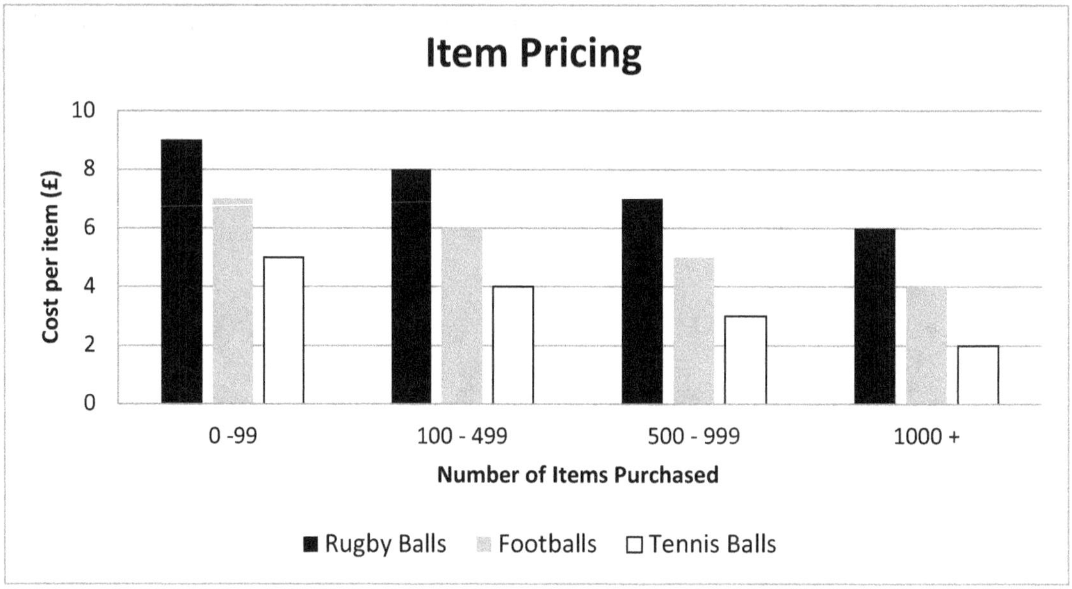

The graph above shows item pricing from a wholesaler. The wholesaler is happy to deliver for a cost of £35 to companies or £5 to individuals. Any order over the cost of £100 qualifies for free delivery. Items are defined as how they come to the wholesaler therefore 1 item = 2 rugby balls or 1 football or 5 tennis balls.

Question 13:
What is the total cost to an individual purchasing 12 rugby balls and 120 tennis balls?

A) £174 B) £179 C) £208 D) £534 E) £588

Question 14:
A private gym wishes to purchase 10 of everything, how short are they of the free delivery boundary?

A) £5.00
B) £5.01
C) £10.00
D) £10.01
E) They are already over the minimum

Question 15:
What is the most number of balls that can be bought by an individual with £1,000 pounds.

A) 200 B) 250 C) 500 D) 1,000 E) 1,250

Question 16:
The wholesaler sells all his products for a profit of 120%. If he sells £1,320 worth of goods at his prices, what did he spend on acquiring them himself?

A) £400 B) £600 C) £800 D) £1,100 E) £1,120

Question 17:
If the wholesaler pays 25% tax on the amount over £12,000 pounds; how much tax does he pay when receiving an order of 2,000 of each item?

A) £2,000 B) £3,000 C) £4,000 D) £5,000 E) £6,000

Question 18:

There are four houses on a street. Lucy, Vicky, and Shannon live in adjacent houses. Shannon has a black dog named Chrissie, Lucy has a white Persian cat and Vicky has a red parrot that shouts obscenities. The owner of a four-legged pet has a blue door. Vicky has a neighbour with a red door. Either a cat or bird owner has a white door. Lucy lives opposite a green door. Vicky and Shannon are not neighbours. What colour is Lucy's door?

A) Green
B) Red
C) White
D) Blue
E) Cannot tell

Question 19:

A train driver runs a service between Cardiff and Merthyr. On average a one-way trip takes 40 minutes to drive but he requires 5 minutes to unload passengers and a further 5 minutes to pick up new ones. As the crow flies the distance between Cardiff and Merthyr is 22 miles.

Assuming he works an 8-hour shift with two 20-minute breaks, and when he arrives to work the first train is already loaded with passengers how far does he travel?

A) 132 B) 143 C) 154 D) 176 E) 198

Question 20:

The massive volume of traffic that travels down the M4 corridor regularly leads to congestion at times of commute morning and evening. A case is being made by local councils in congestion areas to introduce relief lanes thus widening the motorway in an attempt to relieve the congestion. This would involve introducing either a new 2 or 4 lanes to the motorway on average costing 1 million pound per lane per 10 miles.

Many conservationist groups are concerned as this will involve the destruction of large areas of countryside either side of the motorway. They argue that the side of a motorway is a unique habitat with many rare species residing there.

The local councils argue that with many hundreds if not thousands of cars siding idle on the motorway pumping pollutants out into the surrounding areas, it is better for the wildlife if the congestion is eased and traffic can flow through. The councils have also remarked that if congestion is eased there would be less money needed to repair the roads from car incidents with could in theory be given to the conservationist groups as a grant.

Which of the following is assumed in this passage?

A) Wildlife living on the side of the motorway cannot be re-homed.
B) Congestion causes car incidents.
C) Relief lanes have been proven to improve traffic jams.
D) A and B.
E) B and C.
F) All of the above.
G) None of the above.

Question 21:
Who painted *The Nights Watch?*

A) Johannes Vermeer
B) Caravaggio
C) Gian Lorenzo Bernini
D) Rembrandt
E) Peter Paul Rubens

Question 22:
Where did the Japanese nuclear disaster of 2011 occur?

A) Fukushima
B) Hokkaido
C) Tokyo
D) Kyoto
E) Okinawa

END OF SECTION

Section 2

Question 23:
GLUT2 is an essential, ATP independent, mediator in the liver's uptake of plasma glucose. This is an example of:

A) Active transport
B) Diffusion
C) Exocytosis
D) Facilitated Diffusion
E) Osmosis

Question 24:
Which of the following cell types will have the greatest flux along endocytotic pathways?

A) Kidney cells
B) Liver cells
C) Nerve cells
D) Red blood cells
E) White blood cell

Question 25:
Compared to the Krebs cycle, the Calvin cycle demonstrates which of the following differences?

A) CO_2 as a substrate rather than a product
B) Photon dependent
C) Utilisation of different electron transporters
D) Net loss of ATP
E) All of the above

Question 26:
Pepsin and trypsin are both digestive enzymes. Pepsin acts in the stomach whereas trypsin is secreted by the pancreas. Which graph below (trypsin in black and pepsin in grey) would most accurately demonstrate their relative activity against pH?

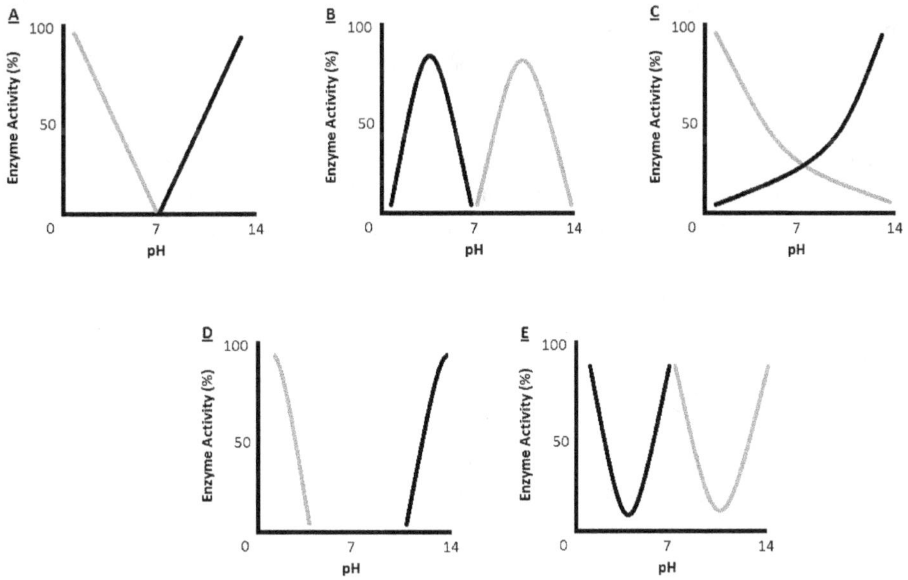

Question 27:
MRSA is an example of:

A) Natural selection
B) Genetic engineering
C) Sexual reproduction
D) Lamarckism
E) Co-dominance

Question 28:
Which of the following statements are correct regarding mitosis?

1. It is important in sexual reproduction.
2. A single round of mitosis results in the formation of 2 genetically distinct daughter cells.
3. Mitosis is vital for tissue growth, as it is the basis for cell multiplication.

A) Only 1
B) Only 2
C) Only 3
D) 1 and 2
E) 2 and 3
F) 1 and 3
G) 1, 2 and 3

Question 29:
Which of the following is the best definition of a mutation?

A) A mutation is a permanent change in DNA.
B) A mutation is a permanent change in DNA that is harmful to an organism.
C) A mutation is a permanent change in the structure of intra-cellular organelles caused by changes in DNA/RNA.
D) A mutation is a permanent change in chromosomal structure caused by DNA/RNA changes.

Question 30:
In relation to mutations, which of the following are correct?

1. Mutations always lead to discernible changes in the phenotype of an organism.
2. Mutations are central to natural processes such as evolution.
3. Mutations play a role in cancer.

A) Only 1
B) Only 2
C) Only 3
D) 1 and 2
E) 2 and 3
F) 1 and 3
G) 1, 2 and 3

Question 31:
Which of the following is the most accurate definition of an antibody?

A) An antibody is a molecule that protects red blood cells from changes in pH.
B) An antibody is a molecule produced only by humans and has a pivotal role in the immune system.
C) An antibody is a toxin produced by a pathogen to damage the host organism.
D) An antibody is a molecule that is used by the immune system to identify and neutralize foreign objects and molecules.
E) Antibodies are small proteins found in red blood cells that help increase oxygen carriage.

Question 32:
Which of the following statements about the kidney are correct?

1. The kidneys filter the blood and remove waste products from the body.
2. The kidneys are involved in the digestion of food.
3. In a healthy individual, the kidneys produce urine that contains high levels of glucose.

A) Only 1
B) Only 2
C) Only 3
D) 1 and 2
E) 2 and 3
F) 1 and 3
G) 1, 2 and 3

Question 33:
Which of the following statements are correct?

1. Hormones are slower acting than nerves.
2. Hormones act for a very short time.
3. Hormones act more generally than nerves.
4. Hormones are released when you get a scare.

A) 1 only
B) 1 and 3 only
C) 2 and 4 only
D) 1, 3 and 4 only
E) 1, 2, 3 and 4

Question 34:
Which statements about homeostasis are correct?

1. Homeostasis is about ensuring the inputs within your body exceed the outputs to maintain a constant internal environment.
2. Homeostasis is about ensuring the inputs within your body are less than the outputs to maintain a constant internal environment.
3. Homeostasis is about balancing the inputs within your body with the outputs to ensure your body fluctuates with the needs of the external environment.
4. Homeostasis is about balancing the inputs within your body with the outputs to maintain a constant internal environment.

A) 1 only
B) 2 only
C) 3 only
D) 4 only
E) 1 and 3 only
F) 2 and 4 only
G) 2 and 3 only

Question 35:

Which of the following statement is true?

A) There is more energy and biomass each time you move up a trophic level.
B) There is less energy and biomass each time you move up a trophic level.
C) There is more energy but less biomass each time you move up a trophic level.
D) There is less energy but more biomass each time you move up a trophic level.
E) There is no difference in the energy or biomass when you move up a trophic level.

Question 36:
Which of the following statements are true about asexual reproduction?

1. There is no fusion of gametes.
2. There are two parents.
3. There is no mixing of chromosomes.
4. There is genetic variation.

A) 1 and 3 only
B) 1 and 4 only
C) 2 and 3 only
D) 3 and 4 only
E) 2 and 4 only
F) 1, 2, 3 and 4

Question 37:

Put the following in the order which they occur when Jonas sees a bowl of chicken and moves towards it.

1. Retina
2. Motor neuron
3. Sensory neuron
4. Brain
5. Muscle

A) 1 - 3 - 4 - 5 - 2
B) 1 - 2 - 3 - 4 - 5
C) 5 - 1 - 3 - 2 - 4
D) 1 - 3 - 2 - 4 - 5
E) 1 - 3 - 4 - 2 - 5
F) 4 - 1 - 3 - 2 - 5

Question 38:

What path does blood take from the kidney to the liver?

1. Pulmonary artery
2. Inferior vena cava
3. Hepatic artery
4. Aorta
5. Pulmonary vein
6. Renal vein

A) 2 - 1 - 4 - 3 - 5 - 6
B) 1 - 2 - 3 - 4 - 5 - 6
C) 6 - 2 - 5 - 1 - 4 - 3
D) 6 - 2 - 1 - 5 - 4 - 3
E) 3 - 2 - 1 - 4 - 6 - 5
F) 3 - 6 - 2 - 4 - 1 – 5

Question 39:

Which of the following statements are true about animal cloning?

1. Animals cloned from embryo transplants are genetically identical.
2. The genetic material is removed from an unfertilised egg during adult cell cloning.
3. Cloning can cause a reduced gene pool.
4. Cloning is only possible with mammals.

A) 1 only
B) 2 only
C) 3 only
D) 4 only
E) 1 and 2 only
F) 1, 2 and 3 only
G) 1, 2, 3 and 4

Question 40:

Which of the following statements are true with regard to evolution?

1. Individuals within a species show variation because of differences in their genes.
2. Beneficial mutations will accumulate within a population.
3. Gene differences are caused by sexual reproduction and mutations.
4. Species with similar characteristics never have similar genes.

A) 1 only
B) 1 and 4 only
C) 2 and 3 only
D) 2 and 4 only
E) 3 and 4 only
F) 1, 2 and 3 only

END OF SECTION

Section 3

Question 41:
The molecular weight of glucose is 180 g/mol. 5.76Kg of glucose is split evenly between two cell cultures under anaerobic conditions. One cell culture is taken from human cardiac muscle, whilst the other is a yeast culture. What will be the difference (in moles) between the amount of CO_2 produced between the two cultures?

A) 0 mol B) 4 mol C) 8 mol D) 12 mol E) 16 mol

Question 42:
What is the electron configuration of magnesium in $MgCl_2$?

A) 2,8
B) 2,8,2
C) 2,8,4
D) 2,8,8
E) None of the above

Question 43:
A calcium sample is run in a mass spectrometer. It is later discovered that the sample was contaminated with the most abundant isotope of chromium. A section of the trace is shown below. What was the actual abundance of the most common calcium isotope?

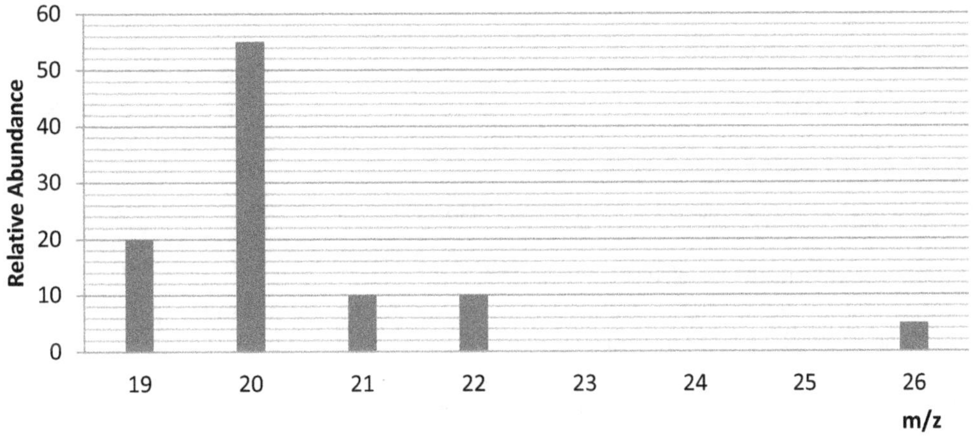

A) 1/9 B) 6/17 C) 1/2 D) 11/19 E) 17/19

Question 44:
A warehouse receives 15 tonnes of arsenic in bulk. Assuming that the sample is at least 80% pure, what is the minimum amount, in moles, of arsenic that they have obtained?

A) 1.6×10^5 B) 2×10^5 C) 1.6×10^6 D) 2×10^6 E) 1.6×10^7

Question 45:
A sample of silicon is run in a mass spectrometer. The resultant trace shows m/z peaks at 26 and 30 with relative abundance 60% and 30% respectively. What other isotope of silicon must have been in the sample to give an average atomic mass of 28?

A) 28 B) 30 C) 32 D) 34 E) 36

Question 46:

72.9g of pure magnesium ribbon is mixed in a reaction vessel with the equivalent of 54g of steam. The ensuing reaction produces $72dm^3$ of hydrogen. Which of the following statements is true?

A) This is a complete reaction
B) This is a partial reaction
C) There is an excess of steam
D) There is an excess of magnesium
E) Magnesium hydroxide is a product

Question 47:

Which species is the reducing agent in: $3Cu^{2+} + 3S^{2-} + 8H^+ + 8NO_3^- \rightarrow 3Cu^{2+} + 3SO_4^{2-} + 8NO + 4H_2O$

A) Cu^{2+} B) S^{2-} C) H^+ D) NO_3^- E) H_2O

Question 48:

Which of the following is not true of alkanes?

A) C_nH2_{n+2}
B) Saturated
C) Reactive
D) Produce only CO_2 and water when burnt in an excess of oxygen
E) None of the above

Question 49:

What values of **s**, **t** and **u** are needed to balance the equation below?

s$AgNO_3$ + **t**$K_3PO_4 \rightarrow 3Ag_3PO_4$ + **u**KNO_3

A) s = 9 t = 3 u = 9
B) s = 6 t = 3 u = 9
C) s = 9 t = 3 u = 6
D) s = 9 t = 6 u = 9
E) s = 3 t = 3 u = 9
F) s = 9 t = 3 u = 3

Question 50:

Which of the following statements are true with regard to displacement?

1. A less reactive halogen can displace a more reactive halogen.
2. Chlorine cannot displace bromine or iodine from an aqueous solution of its salts.
3. Bromine can displace iodine because of the trend of reactivity.
4. Fluorine can displace chlorine as it is higher up the group.
5. Lithium can displace francium as it is higher up the group.

A) 3 only
B) 5 only
C) 1 and 2 only
D) 3 and 4 only
E) 2 , 3 and 5 only
F) 3, 4 and 5 only

Question 51:

What mass of magnesium oxide is produced when 75g of magnesium is burned in excess oxygen?
Relative Atomic Masses: Mg = 24, O = 16

A) 80g B) 100g C) 125g D) 145g E) 175g F) 225g

Question 52:

Hydrogen can combine with hydroxide ions to produce water. Which process is involved in this?

A) Hydration
B) Oxidation
C) Reduction
D) Dehydration
E) Evaporation
F) Precipitation

END OF SECTION

Section 4

Question 53:
A rubber balloon is inflated and rubbed against a sample of animal fur for a period of 15 seconds. At the end of this process the balloon is carrying a charge of -5 coulombs. What magnitude of current must have been induced during the process of rubbing the balloon against the animal fur; and in which direction was it flowing?

A) 0.33A into the balloon
B) 0.33A into the fur
C) 0.33A in no net direction
D) 75A into the balloon
E) 75A into the fur

Question 54:
Which of the following is a unit equivalent to the Amp?

A) V.Ω B) (W.V)/s C) C.Ω D) $(J.s^{-1})/V$ E) C.s

Question 55:
The output of a step-down transformer is measured at 24V and 10A. Given that the transformer is 80% efficient what must the initial power input have been?

A) 240W B) 260W C) 280W D) 300W E) 320W

Question 56:
An electric winch system hoists a mass of 20kg 30 metres into the air over a period of 20 seconds. What is the power output of the winch assuming the system is 100% efficient?

A) 100W B) 200W C) 300W D) 400W E) 500W

Question 57:
6×10^{10} atoms of a radioactive substance remain. The activity of the substance is quantified as 3.6×10^9. What is the decay constant of this material?

A) 0.00006 B) 0.0006 C) 0.006 D) 0.06 E) 0.6

Question 58:
An 80W filament bulb draws 0.5A of household electricity. What is the efficiency of the bulb?

A) 25% B) 33% C) 50% D) 66% E) 75%

Question 59:
An investment of £500 is made in a compound interest account. At the end of 3 years the balance reads £1687.50. What is the interest rate?

A) 20% B) 35% C) 50% D) 65% E) 80%

Question 60:

Rearrange the following equation in terms of t: $x = \frac{\sqrt{b^3-9st}}{13j} + \int_{-z}^{z} 9a - 7$

A) $t = \frac{(13jx - \int_{-z}^{z} 9a-7)^2 - b^3}{9s}$

B) $t = \frac{13jx^2}{b^3-9s} - \int_{-z}^{z} 9a - 7$

C) $t = x - \frac{\sqrt{b^3-9s}}{13j} - \int_{-z}^{z} 9a - 7$

D) $t = \frac{x^2}{\frac{b^3-9s}{13j} + \int_{-z}^{z} 9a-7}$

E) $t = \frac{[13j(x - \int_{-z}^{z} 9a-7)]^2 - b^3}{-9s}$

END OF PAPER

MOCK PAPER C

Section 1

Question 1:
Adam, Beth and Charlie are going on holiday together. A single room costs £60 per night, a double room costs £105 per night and a four-person room costs £215 per night. It is possible to opt out from the cleaning service and to pay £12 less each night per room.

What is the minimum amount the three friends could pay for their holiday for a three-night stay at the hotel?

A) £122 B) £144 C) £203 D) £423 E) £432

Question 2:
I have two 96ml glasses of squash. The first is comprised of $\frac{1}{6}$ squash and $\frac{5}{6}$ water. The second is comprised of $\frac{1}{4}$ water and $\frac{3}{4}$ squash. I take 48ml from the first glass and add it to glass two. I then take 72ml from glass two and add it to glass one.

How much squash is now in each glass?

A) 16ml squash in glass one and 72ml squash in glass two.
B) 40ml squash in glass one and 32ml squash in glass two.
C) 48ml squash in glass one and 32ml squash in glass two.
D) 48ml squash in glass one and 40ml squash in glass two.
E) 80ml squash in glass one and 40ml squash in glass two.

Question 3:
It may amount to millions of pounds each year of taxpayers' money; however, it is strongly advisable for the HPV vaccination in schools to remain. The vaccine, given to teenage girls, has the potential to significantly reduce cervical cancer deaths and furthermore, the vaccines will decrease the requirement for biopsies and invasive procedures related to the follow-up tests. Extensive clinical trials and continued monitoring suggest that both Gardasil and Cervarix are safe and tolerated well by recipients. Moreover, studies demonstrate that a large majority of teenage girls and their parents are in support of the vaccine.

Which of the following is the conclusion of the above argument?

A) HPV vaccines are safe and well tolerated
B) It is strongly advisable for the HPV vaccination in schools to remain
C) The HPV vaccine amounts to millions of pounds each year of taxpayers' money
D) The vaccine has the potential to significantly reduce cervical cancer deaths
E) Vaccinations are vital to disease prevention across the population

Question 4:
Anna cycles to school, which takes 30 minutes. James takes the bus, which leaves from the same place as Anna, but 6 minutes later and gets to school at the same time as Anna. It takes the bus 12 minutes to get to the post office, which is 3km away. The speed of the bus is $\frac{5}{4}$ the speed of the bike. One day Anna leaves 4 minutes late.

How far does she get before she is overtaken by the bus?

A) 1.5km B) 2km C) 3km D) 4km E) 6km

Question 5:
The set two maths teacher is trying to work out who needs to be moved up to set one and who to award a certificate at the end of term. The students must fulfil certain criteria:

Reward	Criteria
Move to set one	Attendance over 95%
	Average test mark over 92
	Less than 5% homework handed in late
Awarded a Certificate	Absences below 4%
	Average test mark over 89
	At least 98% homework handed in on time

	Terry	Alex	Bahara	Lucy	Shiv
Attendance %	97	92	97	100	98
Average test mark %	89	93	94	95	86
Homework handed in on time %	96	92	100	96	98

Who would move up a set and who would receive a certificate?

A) Bahara would move up a set and receive a certificate.
B) Bahara and Lucy would move up a set and Bahara would receive a certificate.
C) Bahara, Terry and Lucy would move up a set and Bahara and Shiv would receive a certificate.
D) Lucy would move up a set and Bahara would receive a certificate.
E) Lucy would move up a set and Bahara and Terry would receive a certificate.

Question 6:
18 years ago, A was 25 years younger than B is now. In 21 years time, A will be 28 years older than B was 14 years ago. How old is A now if A is $\frac{5}{6}$B?

A) 27 B) 28 C) 35 D) 42 E) 46

Question 7:
The time now is 10.45am. I am preparing a meal for 16 guests who will arrive tomorrow for afternoon tea. I want to make 3 scones for each guest, which can be baked in batches of 6. Each batch takes 35 minutes to prepare and 25 minutes to cook in the oven and I can start the next batch while the previous batch is in the oven. I also want to make 2 cupcakes for each guest, which can be baked in batches of 8. It takes 15 minutes to prepare the mixture for each batch and 20 minutes to cook them in the oven. I will also make 3 cucumber sandwiches for each guest. 6 cucumber sandwiches take 5 minutes to prepare.

What will the time be when I finish making all the food for tomorrow?

A) 4:35pm B) 5.55pm C) 6:00pm D) 6:05pm E) 7:20pm

Question 8:

Pyramid	Base edge (m)	Volume (m^3)
1	3	33
2	4	64
3	2	8
4	6	120
5	2	8
6	6	120
7	4	64

What is the difference between the height of the smallest and tallest pyramids?

A) 1m B) 5m C) 4m D) 6m E) 8m

Question 9:

At the final stop (stop 6), 10 people get off the tube. At the previous stop (stop 5) $\frac{1}{2}$ of passengers got off. At stop 4, $\frac{3}{5}$ of passengers got off. At stop 3, $\frac{1}{3}$ of passengers got off and at stops 1 and 2, $\frac{1}{6}$ of passengers got off.

How many passengers got on at the first stop?

A) 10 B) 36 C) 90 D) 108 E) 3600

Question 10:

It is important that research universities demonstrate convincing support of teaching. Undergraduates comprise an overwhelming proportion of all students and universities should make an effort to cater to the requirements of the majority of their student body. After all, many of these students may choose to pursue a path involving research and a strong education would provide students with skills equipped towards a career in research.

What is the conclusion of the above argument?

A) Undergraduates comprise an overwhelming proportion of all students.
B) A strong education would provide a strong foundation and skills equipped towards a career in research.
C) Research universities should strongly support teaching.
D) Institutions should provide undergraduates with a high-quality learning experience.
E) Research has a greater impact than teaching and limited universities funds should mainly be invested in research.

Question 11:

American football has reached a level of violence that puts its players at too high a level of risk. It has been suggested that the NFL, the governing body for American football should get rid of the iconic helmets. The hard-plastic helmets all have to meet minimum impact-resistance standards intended to enhance safety, however in reality they gave players a false sense of security that only resulted in harder collisions. Some players now suffer from early onset dementia, mood swings and depression. The proposal to ban helmets for good should be supported. Moreover, it would prevent costly legal settlements involving the NFL and ex-players suffering from head trauma.

What is the conclusion of the above argument?

A) Sports players should not be exposed to unnecessary danger.
B) Helmets give players a false sense of security.
C) Players can suffer from early onset dementia, mood swings and depression.
D) The proposal to ban helmets should be supported.
E) American football is too violent and puts its players at risk.

Question 12:

Everyone likes English. Some students born in spring like Maths and some like Biology. All students born in winter like Music and some like Art. Of those born in autumn, no one likes Biology, and everyone likes Art.

Which of the following is true?

A) Some students born in spring like both Biology and Maths.
B) Students born in spring, winter, and autumn all like Art.
C) No one born in winter or autumn likes Biology.
D) No one who likes Biology also likes Art.
E) Some students born in winter like 3 subjects.

Question 13:

Until the twentieth century, the whole purpose of art was to create beautiful, flawless works. Artists attained a level of skill and craft that took decades to perfect and could not be mirrored by those who had not taken great pains to master it. The serenity and beauty produced from movements such as impressionism has however culminated in repulsive and horrific displays of rotting carcasses designed to provoke an emotional response rather than admiration. These works cannot be described as beautiful by either the public or art critics. While these works may be engaging on an intellectual or academic level, they no longer constitute art.

Which of the following is an assumption of the above argument?

A) Beauty is a defining property of art.
B) All modern art is ugly.
C) Twenty first century artists do not study for decades.
D) The impressionist movement created beautiful works of art.
E) Some modern art provokes an emotional response.

Question 14:
The cost of sunglasses is reduced over the bank holiday weekend. On Saturday, the price of the sunglasses on Friday is reduced by 10%. On Sunday the price of the sunglasses on Saturday is reduced by 10%. On Monday, the price of the sunglasses on Sunday is reduced by a further 10%. What percentage of the price on Friday is the price of the sunglasses on Monday?

A) 55.12% B) 59.10% C) 63.80% D) 70.34% E) 72.9%

Question 15:
When folded, which box can be made from the net shown below?

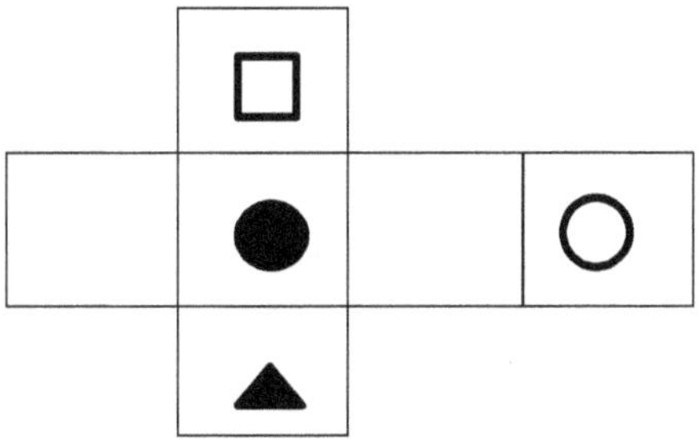

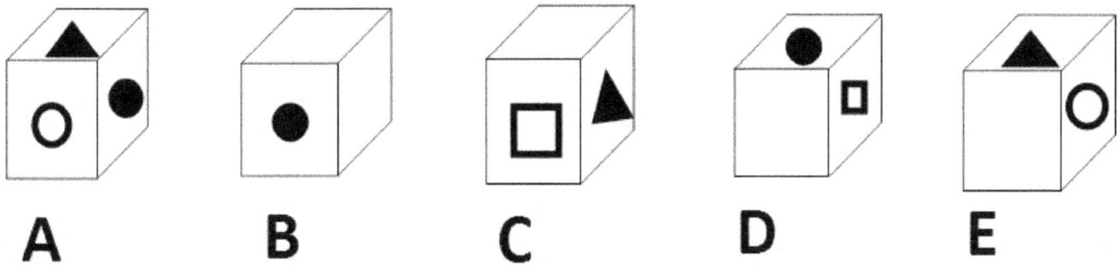

Questions 16-18 refer to the following information:

$$BMI = weight\ (kg)\ \div\ height^2\ (m^2)$$

Men	**BMR= (10 x weight in kg) + (6.25 x height in cm) – (5 x age in years) + 5**
Women	**BMR= (10 x weight in kg) + (6.25 x height in cm) – (5 x age in years) -161**

Recommended Intake:

Amount of Exercise	Daily Kilocalories required
Little to no exercise	BMR x 1.2
Light exercise 1-3 days per week	BMR x 1.375
Moderate exercise 3-5 days per week	BMR x 1.55
Heavy exercise 6-7 days per week	BMR x 1.725
Very heavy exercise twice per day	BMR x 1.9

Question 16:
A child weighs 35kg and is 120cm tall. What is the BMI of the child to the nearest two decimal places?

A) 0.0024 B) 24.28 C) 24.31 D) 42.01 E) 42.33

Question 17:
What is the BMR of a 32-year-old woman weighing 80kg and measuring 1.7m in height?

A) 643.7 kcal B) 1537 kcal C) 1541.5 kcal D) 1707.5 kcal E) 2707.5 kcal

Question 18:
What is the recommended intake of a 45-year-old man weighing 80kg and measuring 1.7m in height who does little to no exercise each week?

A) 1642.5 kcal B) 1771.8 kcal C) 1851 kcal D) 1971 kcal E) 2712.5 kcal

Question 19:
Putting the digit 7 on the right-hand side of a two-digit number causes the number to increase by 565. What is the value of the two-digit number?

A) 27 B) 52 C) 62 D) 66 E) 627

Question 20:
The grid is comprised of 49 squares. The shape's area is $588cm^2$. What is its perimeter in cm?

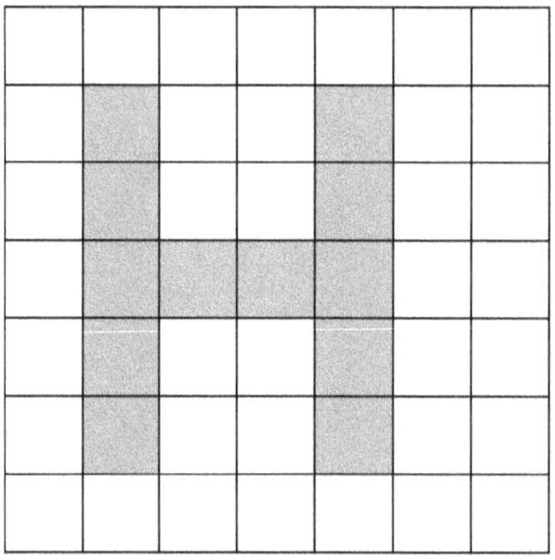

A) 26 B) 49 C) 84 D) 126 E) 182

Question 21:
Which UN organisation motto is *'foster global monetary cooperation, secure financial stability, facilitate international trade, promote high employment and sustainable economic growth, and reduce poverty around the world'*

A) FAO B) WTO C) IMF D) WHO E) IFAD

Question 22:
Which building does not match the city it is in

A) Paris – Arc de Triomph
B) Madrid – Temple of Debod
C) Stockholm – Storkyrkan
D) Moscow – Cathedral of Christ the Saviour
E) Berlin – Schonbrunn Palace

END OF SECTION

Section 2

Question 23:
Which of the following statements regarding enzymes are correct?

1. Enzymes are denatured at high temperatures or extreme pH values.
2. Amylase is produced in the salivary glands only and converts starch to sugars.
3. Lipases catalyse the breakdown of oils and fats into glycerol and fatty acids. This takes place in the small intestine.
4. Bile is stored in the pancreas and travels down the bile duct to neutralise stomach acid.
5. Isomerase can be used to convert glucose into fructose for use in slimming products.

A) 1 and 3 only
B) 1, 3 and 4 only
C) 1, 3 and 5
D) 2 and 4 only
E) 3 and 5 only

Question 24:
Which of the following describes the role of the colon?

A) Food is combined with bile and digestive enzymes.
B) Storage of faeces.
C) Reabsorption of water.
D) Faeces leave the alimentary canal.
E) Any digested food is absorbed into the lymph and blood.

Question 25:
Which of the following are true?

1. A nerve impulse is transmitted along the nerve axon as an electrical impulse and across the synapse by diffusion of chemical neurotransmitters.
2. Drugs that block synaptic transmission can cause complete paralysis.
3. The fatty sheath around the axon slows the speed at which nerve impulses are transmitted.
4. The peripheral nervous system includes the brain and spinal cord.
5. A reflex arc bypasses the brain and enables a fast, autonomic response.

A) 1 and 2
B) 1, 2 and 3
C) 1, 2 and 5
D) 2, 4 and 5
E) 3, 4 and 5

Question 26:
Which of the following statements regarding the circulatory system are correct?

1. The pulmonary artery carries oxygenated blood from the right ventricle to the lungs.
2. The aorta has a high content of elastic tissue and carries oxygenated blood from the left ventricle around the body.
3. The mitral valve is between the pulmonary vein and the left atrium.
4. The vena cava carries deoxygenated blood from the body to the right atrium.

A) 1 and 3 B) 1 and 2 C) 2 only D) 2 and 4 E) 3 only

Question 27:

Tongue-rolling is controlled by the dominant allele T, while non-rolling is controlled by the recessive allele, t. Red-green colour blindness is controlled by a sex-linked gene on the X chromosome. Normal colour vision is controlled by dominant allele B, while red-green colour blindness is controlled by the recessive allele, b. The mother of a family is colour blind and heterozygous for tongue-rolling, while the father has normal colour vision and is a non-roller.

Which of the following statements are correct?

1. More males than females in a population are red-green colour blind.
2. 50% of children will be non-rollers.
3. All the male children will be colour-blind.

A) 1 and 2 only
B) 1, 2 and 3
C) 2 only
D) 2 and 3 only
E) 3 only

Question 28:

Which of the following are true?

1. Lightning, as well as nitrogen-fixing bacteria, converts nitrogen gas to nitrate compounds.
2. Decomposers return nitrogen to the soil as ammonia.
3. The shells of marine animals contain calcium carbonate, which is derived from dietary carbon.
4. Nitrogen is used to make the amino acids found in proteins.

A) 1 only
B) 1 and 2
C) 2 and 3
D) 2, 3 and 4
E) They are all true

Question 29:

Which of the following are correct regarding polymers?

1. Sucrose is formed by the condensation of hundreds of monosaccharides.
2. Lactose is found in milk and is formed by condensation of two glucose molecules.
3. Glucose has two isomers.
4. Glycogen, starch and cellulose are all polysaccharides formed by condensation of multiple glucose molecules.
5. People with lactose intolerance lack lactase and can experience diarrhoea after drinking milk.

A) 1 only
B) 1, 2 and 3
C) 1 and 3 only
D) 3, 4 and 5
E) 4 and 5 only

Question 30:

Which of the following genetic statements are correct?

1. Alleles are a similar version of different cells.
2. If you are homozygous for a trait, you have three alleles the same for that particular gene.
3. If you are heterozygous for a trait, you have two different alleles for that particular gene.
4. To show the characteristic that is caused by a recessive allele, both carried alleles for the gene have to be recessive.

A) 1 only
B) 2 only
C) 3 only
D) 4 only
E) 1 and 2 only
F) 3 and 4 only
G) 1, 2, and 3 only

Question 31:
Which of the following statements are correct about meiosis?

1. The DNA content of a gamete is half that of a human red blood cell.
2. Meiosis requires ATP.
3. Meiosis only takes place in reproductive tissue.
4. In meiosis, a diploid cell divides in such a way so as to produce two haploid cells.

A) 1 only
B) 3 only
C) 1 and 2 only
D) 2 and 3 only
E) 2 and 4 only
F) 1, 2, 3 and 4

Question 32:
Put the following statements in the correct order of events for when there is too little water in the blood.

1. Urine is more concentrated
2. Pituary gland releases ADH
3. Blood water level returns to normal
4. Hypothalamus detects too little water in blood
5. Kidney affects water level

A) 1 - 2 - 3 - 4 - 5
B) 5 - 4 - 3 - 2 - 1
C) 4 - 2 - 5 - 1 - 3
D) 3 - 2 - 4 - 1 - 5
E) 5 - 2 - 3 - 4 - 1
F) 4 - 2 – 1- 5 - 3

Question 33:
The pH of venous blood is 7.35. Which of the following is the likely pH of arterial blood?

A) 4.4
B) 5.2
C) 6.5
D) 7.0
E) 7.4
F) 7.95

Question 34:
Which of the following are true of the cytoplasm?

1. The vast majority of the cytoplasm is made up of water.
2. All contents of animal cells are contained in the cytoplasm.
3. The cytoplasm contains electrolytes and proteins.

A) 1 only
B) 2 only
C) 3 only
D) 1 and 2 only
E) 1 and 3 only
F) 1, 2 and 3

Question 35:
ATP is produced in which of the following organelles?

1. The golgi apparatus
2. The rough endoplasmic reticulum
3. The mitochondria
4. The nucleus

A) 1 only
B) 2 only
C) 3 only
D) 4 only
E) 1 and 2
F) 2 and 3 only
G) 3 and 4 only
H) 1, 2, 3 and 4

Question 36:

The cell membrane:

A) Is made up of a phospholipid bilayer which only allows active transport across it.
B) Is not found in bacteria.
C) Is a semi-permeable barrier to ions and organic molecules.
D) Consists purely of enzymes.

Question 37:

Cells of the *Polyommatus atlantica* butterfly of the Lycaenidae family have 446 chromosomes. Which of the following statements about a *P. atlantica* butterfly are correct?

1. Mitosis will produce 2 daughter cells each with 223 pairs of chromosomes
2. Meiosis will produce 4 daughter cells each with 223 chromosomes
3. Mitosis will produce 4 daughter cells each with 446 chromosomes
4. Meiosis will produce 2 daughter cells each with 223 pairs of chromosomes

A) 1 and 2 only
B) 1 and 3 only
C) 2 and 3 only
D) 3 and 4 only
E) 1, 2 and 3 only
F) 1, 2, 3 and 4

Questions 38-40 are based on the following information:

Assume that hair colour is determined by a single allele. The R allele is dominant and results in black hair. The r allele is recessive for red hair. Mary (red hair) and Bob (black hair) are having a baby girl.

Question 38:

What is the probability that she will have red hair?

A) 0% only
B) 25% only
C) 50% only
D) 0% or 25%
E) 0% or 50%
F) 25% or 50%

Question 39:

Mary and Bob have a second child, Tim, who is born with red hair. What does this confirm about Bob?

A) Bob is heterozygous for the hair allele.
B) Bob is homozygous dominant for the hair allele.
C) Bob is homozygous recessive for the hair allele.
D) Bob does not have the hair allele.

Question 40:

Mary and Bob go on to have a third child. What are the chances that this child will be born homozygous for black hair?

A) 0%
B) 25%
C) 50%
D) 75%
E) 100%

END OF SECTION

Section 3

Question 41:

Which of the following statements are true regarding the transition elements?

1. Iron (II) compounds are light green.
2. Transition elements are neither malleable nor ductile.
3. Transition metal carbonates may undergo thermal decomposition.
4. Transition metal hydroxides are soluble in water.
5. When Cu^{2+} ions are mixed with sodium hydroxide solution, a blue precipitate is formed.

A) 1 and 2 B) 1 and 3 C) 1, 3 and 5 D) 3 and 5 E) 5 only

Question 42:

What is the value of C when the equation is balanced?

<u>*5*</u> $PhCH_3$ + <u>*A*</u> $KMnO_4$ + <u>*9*</u> H_2SO_4 = <u>*5*</u> PhCOOH + <u>***B***</u> K_2SO_4 + <u>***C***</u> $MnSO_4$ + <u>*14*</u> H_2O

A) 3 B) 4 C) 5 D) 7 E) 9

Question 43:

What is the mass in grams of calcium chloride, $CaCl_2$, in 25cm^3 of a solution with a concentration of 0.1 mol.l^{-1}? (Ar of Ca is 40 and Ar of Cl is 35)

A) 0.28g B) 0.46g C) 0.48g D) 0.72g E) 1.28g

Question 44:

16.4g of nitrobenzene is produced from 13g of benzene in excess nitric acid: $C_6H_6 + HNO_3 \rightarrow C_6H_5NO_2 + H_2O$

What is the percentage yield of nitrobenzene ($C_6H_5NO_2$)?

A) 65% B) 67% C) 72% D) 78% E) 80%

Question 45:

Which of the following statements are false?

1. Simple molecules do not conduct electricity because there are no free electrons and there is no overall charge.
2. The carbon and silicon atoms in silica are arranged in a giant lattice structure and it has a very high melting point.
3. Ionic compounds do not conduct electricity when dissolved in water or when melted because the ions are too far apart.
4. Alloys are harder than pure metals.

A) 1 and 2 C) 1, 2, 3 and 4 E) 3 only

B) 1, 2 and 4 D) 2 and 4

Question 46:

A compound with a molar mass of 120 g.mol^{-1} contains 12g of carbon, 2g of hydrogen and 16g oxygen. What is the molecular formula of the compound?

A) CH_2O B) $C_2H_4O_2$ C) C_4H_2O D) $C_4H_8O_4$ E) $C_8H_{16}O_8$

Question 47:
The following points refer to the halogens:

1. Iodine is a grey solid and can be used to sterilise wounds. It forms a purple vapour when warmed.
2. The melting and boiling points increase as you go up the group.
3. Fluorine is very dangerous and reacts instantly with iron wool, whereas iodine must be strongly heated as well as the iron wool for a reaction to occur and the reaction is slow.
4. When bromine is added to sodium chloride, the bromine displaces chlorine from sodium chloride.
5. The hydrogen atom and chlorine atom in hydrogen chloride are joined by a covalent bond.

Which of the above statements are false?

A) 1, 3 and 5
B) 1, 2 and 3
C) 2 and 4
D) 3 only
E) 3, 4 and 5

Question 48:
Which of the following statements about Ammonia are correct?

1. It has a formula of NH_3.
2. Nitrogen contributes 82% to its mass.
3. It can be broken down again into nitrogen and hydrogen.
4. It is covalently bonded.
5. It is used to make fertilisers.

A) 1 and 2 only
B) 1 and 4 only
C) 1, 2 and 3 only
D) 1, 2 and 5 only
E) 3, 4 and 5 only
F) 1, 2, 3, 4 and 5

Question 49:
What colour will a universal indicator change to in a solution of milk and lipase?

A) From green to orange.
B) From red to green.
C) From purple to green.
D) From purple to orange.
E) From yellow to purple.
F) From purple to red.

Question 50:
Vitamin C [$C_6H_8O_6$] can be artificially synthesised from glucose [$C_6H_{12}O_6$]. What type of reaction is this likely to be?

A) Dehydration
B) Hydration
C) Oxidation
D) Reduction
E) Displacement
F) Evaporation

Question 51:
Which of the following statements are true?

1. Cu^{64} will undergo oxidation faster than Cu^{65}.
2. Cu^{65} will undergo reduction faster than Cu^{64}.
3. Cu^{65} and Cu^{64}have the same number of electrons.

A) 1 only
B) 2 only
C) 3 only
D) 2 and 3 only
E) 1 and 3 only
F) 1, 2 and 3

Question 52:

6g of Mg^{24} is added to a solution containing 30g of dissolved sulphuric acid (H_2SO_4). Which of the following statements are true?

Relative Atomic Masses: S = 32, Mg = 24, O = 16, H = 1

1. In this reaction, the magnesium is the limiting reagent
2. In this reaction, sulphuric acid is the limiting reagent
3. The mass of salt produced equals the original mass of sulphuric acid

A) 1 only
B) 2 only
C) 3 only
D) 1 and 2 only
E) 1 and 3 only
F) 2 and 3 only

END OF SECTION

Section 4

Question 53:

Make *y* the subject of the formula: $\frac{y+x}{x} = \frac{x}{a} + \frac{a}{x}$

A) $y = \frac{x^2}{a} + a$

B) $y = \frac{x^2+a^2-ax}{a}$

C) $y = \frac{-ax}{x^2+a^2}$

D) $y = \frac{x^2}{ax} + a - x$

E) $y = a^2 - ax$

Question 54:

Consider the equations: A: y = 3x and B: $y = \frac{6}{x} - 7$. At what values of x do the two equations intersect?

A) x=2 and x=9
B) x=3 and x=6
C) x=6 and x=27
D) x=6
E) x=18

Question 55:

Rupert plays one game of tennis and one game of squash.
The probability that he will win the tennis game is $\frac{3}{4}$
The probability that he will win the squash game is $\frac{1}{3}$
What is the probability that he will win one game only?

A) $\frac{3}{12}$ B) $\frac{7}{12}$ C) $\frac{4}{5}$ D) $\frac{13}{12}$ E) $\frac{7}{6}$

Question 56:

What is the median of the following numbers: $\frac{7}{36}$; $0.\dot{3}$; $\frac{11}{18}$; 0.25; 0.75; $\frac{62}{72}$; $\frac{7}{7}$

A) $\frac{7}{36}$ B) $0.\dot{3}$ C) $\frac{11}{18}$ D) $\frac{62}{72}$ E) 0.75

Question 57:

Two carriages of a train collide and then start moving together in the same direction. Carriage 1 has mass 12,000 kg and moves at $5ms^{-1}$ before the collision. Carriage 2 has mass 8,000 kg and is stationary before the collision.
What is the velocity of the two carriages after the collision?

A) $2\ ms^{-1}$ B) $3\ ms^{-1}$ C) $4\ ms^{-1}$ D) $4.5\ ms^{-1}$ E) $5\ ms^{-1}$

Question 58:
Which of the following points regarding electromagnetic waves are correct?

1. Radiowaves have the longest wavelength and the lowest frequency.
2. Infrared has a shorter wavelength than visible light and is used in optical fibre communication, and heater and night vision equipment.
3. All of the waves from gamma to radio waves travel at the speed of light (about 300,000,000 m/s).
4. Infrared radiation is used to sterilise food and to kill cancer cells.
5. Darker skins absorb more UV light, so less ultraviolet radiation reaches the deeper tissues.

A) 1 and 2
B) 1 and 3
C) 1, 3 and 5
D) 2 and 3
E) 2 and 4

Question 59:
Which of the following statements are true?

1. Control rods are used to absorb electrons in a nuclear reactor to control the chain reaction.
2. Nuclear fusion is commonly used as an energy source.
3. An alpha particle is comprised of two protons and two neutrons and is the same as a helium nucleus.
4. When ${}^{14}_{6}C$ undergoes beta decay, an electron and ${}^{14}_{7}N$ are produced.
5. Beta particles are less ionising than gamma rays and more ionising than alpha particles.

A) 1 and 2
B) 1 and 3
C) 3 and 4
D) 3, 4 and 5
E) None

Question 60:
Simplify fully: $\frac{(3x^{1/2})^3}{3x^2}$

A) $\frac{3x}{\sqrt{x}}$
B) $\frac{9}{x}$
C) $3x^{1/2}$
D) $3x\sqrt{x}$
E) $\frac{9}{\sqrt{x}}$

END OF PAPER

MOCK PAPER D

Section 1

Question 1:

"Competitors need to be able to run 200 metres in under 25 seconds to qualify for a tournament. James, Steven and Joe are attempting to qualify. Steven and Joe run faster than James. James' best time over 200 metres is 26.2 seconds." Which response is definitely true?

A) Only Joe qualifies.
B) James does not qualify.
C) Joe and Steven both qualify.
D) Joe qualifies.
E) No one qualifies.

Question 2:

You spend £5.60 in total on a sandwich, a packet of crisps and a watermelon. The watermelon cost twice as much as the sandwich, and the sandwich cost twice the price of the crisps.
How much did the watermelon cost?

A) £1.20
B) £2.60
C) £2.80
D) £3.20
E) £3.60

Question 3:

Jane, Chloe and Sam are all going by train to a football match. Chloe gets the 2:15pm train. Sam's journey takes twice as long Jane's. Sam catches the 3:00pm train. Jane leaves 20 minutes after Chloe and arrives at 3:25pm. When will Sam arrive?

A) 3:50pm
B) 4:10pm
C) 4:15pm
D) 4:30pm
E) 4:40pm

Question 4:

Alex gets a pay rise of 5% plus an extra £6 per week. The flat rate of income tax on his salary is decreased from 14% to 12% at the same time. Alex's old weekly take-home pay after tax is £250 per week.
What will his new weekly take-home pay be, to the nearest whole pound?

A) £260
B) £267
C) £273
D) £279
E) £285

Question 5:

You have four boxes, each containing two cubes. Box A contains two white cubes, Box B contains two black cubes, and Boxes C and D both contain one white cube and one black cube. You pick a box at random and take out one cube. It is a white cube. You then draw another cube from the same box.
What is the probability that this cube is not white?

A) ½
B) ⅓
C) ⅔
D) ¼
E) ¾

Question 6:

Anderson & Co. hire out heavy plant machinery at a cost of £500 per day. There is a surcharge for heavy usage, at a rate of £10 per minute of usage over 80 minutes. Concordia & Co. charge £600 per day for similar machinery, plus £5 for every minute of usage. For what duration of usage are the costs the same for both companies?

A) 100 minutes
B) 130 minutes
C) 140 minutes
D) 170 minutes
E) 180 minutes

Question 7:
Simon is discussing with Seth whether or not a candidate is suitable for a job. When pressed for a weakness at interview, the candidate told Simon that he is a slow eater. Simon argues that this will reduce the candidate's productivity, since he will be inclined to take longer lunch breaks.

Which statement **best** supports Simon's argument?
A) Slow eaters will take longer to eat lunch
B) Longer lunch breaks are a distraction
C) Eating more slowly will reduce the time available to work
D) Eating slowly is a weakness
E) Eating slowly will lead to less time to work efficiently

Question 8:
Three pieces of music are on repeat in different rooms of a house. One piece of music is three minutes long, one is four minutes long and the final one is 100 seconds long. All pieces of music start playing at exactly the same time. How long is it until they are next starting together again?

A) 12 minutes
B) 15 minutes
C) 20 minutes
D) 60 minutes
E) 300 minutes

Question 9:
A car leaves Salisbury at 8:22am and travels 180 miles to Lincoln, arriving at 12:07pm. Near Warwick, the driver stopped for a 14 minute break.
What was its average speed, whilst travelling, in kilometres per hour? It should be assumed that the conversion from miles to kilometres is 1:1.6.

A) 51kph B) 67kph C) 77kph D) 82kph E) 86kph

Questions 10 and 11 refer to the following data:

Five respondents were asked to estimate the value of three bottles of wine, in pounds sterling.

Respondent	Wine 1	Wine 2	Wine 3
1	13	16	25
2	17	16	23
3	11	17	21
4	13	15	14
5	15	19	29
Actual retail value	**8**	**25**	**23**

Question 10:
What is the mean error made when guessing the value of wine 1?

A) £4.80 B) £5.60 C) £5.80 D) £6.20 E) £6.40

Question 11:
Which respondent guessed most accurately?

A) Respondent 1
B) Respondent 2
C) Respondent 3
D) Respondent 4
E) Respondent 5

Question 12:

"Recently in Kansas, a number of farm animals have been found killed in the fields. The nature of the injuries is mysterious, but consistent with tales of alien activity. Local people talk of a number of UFO sightings, and claim extra terrestrial responsibility. Official investigations into these claims have dismissed them, offering rational explanations for the reported phenomena. However, these official investigations have failed to deal with the point that, even if the UFO sightings can be explained in rational terms, the injuries on the carcasses of the farm animals cannot be. Extra terrestrial beings must therefore be responsible for these attacks."

Which of the following best expresses the main conclusion of this argument?

A) Sightings of UFOs cannot be explained by rational means
B) Recent attacks must have been carried out by extraterrestrial beings
C) The injuries on the carcasses are not due to normal predators
D) UFO sightings are common in Kansas
E) Official investigations were a cover-up

Question 13:

"To make a cake you must prepare the ingredients and then bake it in the oven. You purchase the required ingredients from the shop, however your oven is broken. Therefore you cannot make a cake."

Which of the following arguments has the same structure?

A) To get a good job, you must have a strong CV then impress the recruiter at interview. Your CV was not as good as other applicants; therefore you didn't get the job.
B) To get to Paris, you must either fly or take the Eurostar. There are flight delays due to dense fog, therefore you must take the Eurostar.
C) To borrow a library book, you must go to the library and show your library card. At the library, you realise you have forgotten your library card. Therefore you cannot borrow a book.
D) To clean a bedroom window, you need a ladder and a hosepipe. Since you don't have the right equipment, you cannot clean the window.
E) Bears eat both fruit and fish. The river is frozen, so the bear cannot eat fish.

Question 14:

"Making model ships requires patience, skill and experience. Patience and skill without experience is common – but often such people give up prematurely, since skill without experience is insufficient to make model ships, and patience can quickly be exhausted."

Which of the following summarises the main argument?

A) Most people lack the skill needed to make model ships
B) Making model ships requires experience
C) The most important thing is to get experience
D) Most people make model ships for a short time but give up due to a lack of skill
E) Successful model ship makers need to have several positive traits

Question 15:

"Joseph has a bag of building blocks of various shapes and colours. Some of the cubic ones are black. Some of the black ones are pyramid shaped. All blue ones are cylindrical. There is a green one of each shape. There are some pink shapes."

Which of the following is definitely **NOT** true?

A) Joseph has pink cylindrical blocks
B) Joseph doesn't have pink cylindrical blocks
C) Joseph has blue cubic blocks
D) Joseph has a green pyramid
E) Joseph doesn't have a black sphere

Question 16:
A fair 6-faced die has 2 sides painted red. The die is rolled 3 times.
What is the probability that at least one red side has been rolled?

A) $^{8}/_{27}$ B) $^{19}/_{27}$ C) $^{21}/_{27}$ D) $^{24}/_{27}$ E) 1

Question 17:
"In a particular furniture warehouse, all chairs have four legs. No tables have five legs, nor do any have three. Beds have no less than four legs, but one bed has eight as they must have a multiple of four legs. Sofas have four or six legs. Wardrobes have an even number of legs, and sideboards have and odd number. No other furniture has legs. Brian picks a piece of furniture out, and it has six legs."

What can be deduced about this piece of furniture?

A) It is a table
B) It could be either a wardrobe or a sideboard
C) It must be either a table or a sofa
D) It must be either a table, a sofa or a wardrobe
E) It could be either a bed, a table or a sofa

Question 18:
Two friends live 42 miles away from each other. They walk at 3mph towards each other. One of them has a pet falcon which starts to fly at 18mph as soon as the friends set off. The falcon flies back and forth between the two friends until the friends meet. How many miles does the falcon travel in total?

A) 63 B) 84 C) 114 D) 126 E) 252

Question 19:
"Antibiotic resistance is on the increase. As a result, many antibiotics in our vast armoury are becoming ineffective against common infections. Probably the most significant contributor to this is the use of antibiotics in farming, as this exposes bacteria to antibiotics for no good reason, giving the opportunity for resistance to develop. If this worrying trend continues, we might, in 30 years time, be back in the Victorian situation, where people die from skin or chest infections we consider mild today."

Which of the following best represents the overall conclusion of the passage?

A) Antibiotic resistance is a serious issue
B) Antibiotics use in farming is essential
C) The use of antibiotics in farming could cause us serious harm
D) Victorians used to die from diseases we can treat today
E) Antibiotics can treat skin infections

Question 20:
A complete set of maths equipment includes a pen, a pencil, a geometry set and a pad of paper. Pens cost £1.50, pencils cost 50p, paper pads cost £1 and geometry sets cost £3. Sam, Dave and George each want complete sets, but Mr Browett persuades them to share some items. Sam and Dave agree to share a paper pad and a geometry set. George must have his own pen, but agrees that he and Sam can share a pencil.

What is the total amount spent?
A) £12.00 B) £13.50 C) £16.50 D) £17.50 E) £18.00

Question 21:
Who has remained president of Syria during the Arab spring and Syrian civil war?

A) Hosni Mubarak
B) Muammar Gaddafi
C) Bashar al-Assad
D) Zine el Ben Ali
E) Abdullah bin Al-Hussein

Question 22:
Who wrote *Leviathon*?

A) Thomas Hobbes
B) Immanuel Kant
C) Niccolo Machiavelli
D) Rene Descartes
E) Jean-Jacques Rousseau

END OF SECTION

Section 2

Question 23:
Which of the following is **NOT** present in the Bowman's capsule?

A) Urea
B) Glucose
C) Sodium
D) Water
E) Haemoglobin

Question 24:
The primary ions responsible for an action potential on a muscle cell membrane are Sodium and Potassium. Sodium concentration is higher than that of potassium outside the cell. Potassium concentration is higher than that of sodium inside the cell. Depolarisation occurs when the membrane potential increases (become more positive).
Which of the following **must** be true when a muscle cell membrane depolarises?

A) More potassium moves into the muscle cell than sodium.
B) More sodium moves into the muscle cell than potassium.
C) There is no net flow of sodium or potassium ions.
D) The membrane potential becomes more negative
E) None of the above

Question 25:
Which of the following in NOT a polymer?

A) Polythene
B) Glycogen
C) Collagen
D) Starch
E) DNA
F) Triglyceride

Question 26:
SIADH is a metabolic disorder caused by an excess of Anti-Diuretic Hormone (ADH) release by the posterior pituitary gland.

Which row best describes the urine produced by a patient with SIADH?

	Volume	Salt Concentration	Glucose
A)	High	Low	Low
B)	High	High	Low
C)	High	High	High
D)	Low	Low	Low
E)	Low	High	Low
F)	Low	High	High

Question 27:
The normal cardiac cycle has two phases, systole and diastole.

During diastole, which of the following is **FALSE**?
A) The aortic valve is closed
B) The ventricles are relaxing
C) There is blood in the ventricles
D) The pressure in the aorta increases
E) There is blood in the ventricles

Question 28:

Below is a graph showing the concentration of product over time as substrate concentration is increased. Some enzyme inhibitors are introduced.

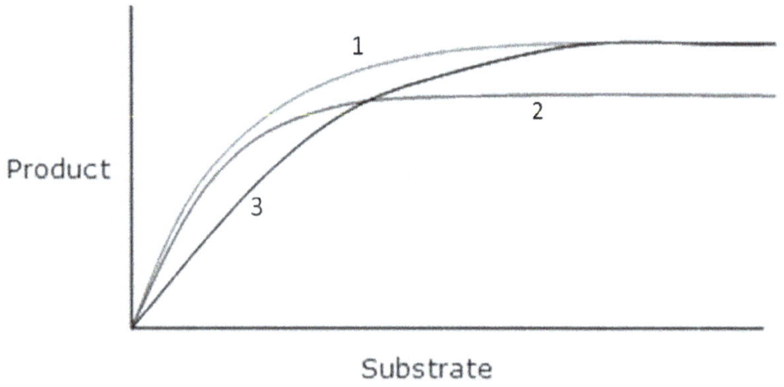

Which, if any, line represents the effect of competitive inhibition?

A) Line 1
B) Line 2
C) Line 3
D) None of these lines

Question 29:

Which of the following is **NOT** present in the plasma membrane?

A) Extrinsic proteins
B) Intrinsic proteins
C) Phospholipids
D) Glycoproteins
E) Nucleic Acids
F) They are all present

Question 30:

A pulmonary embolism occurs when a main artery supplying the lungs becomes blocked by a clot that has travelled from somewhere else in the body.

Which option best describes the path of a blood clot that originated in the leg and has caused a pulmonary embolism?

A. Inferior Vena cava
B. Superior Vena cava
C. Right atrium
D. Right ventricle
E. Left atrium
F. Left ventricle
G. Pulmonary artery
H. Pulmonary vein
I. Aorta
J. Coronary artery

A) C, D, H, G
B) B, C, D, H, G
C) I, E, F, G
D) A, C, D, G
E) A, C, D, J, G
F) A, C, D, J, E, F, G

Question 31:
The concentration of chloride in the blood is 100mM. The concentration of thyroxine is 1×10^{-10}kM. Calculate the ratio of thyroxine to chloride ions in the blood.

A) Chloride is 100,000,000 times more concentrated than thyroxine
B) Chloride is 1,000,000 times more concentrated than thyroxine
C) Chloride is 1000 times more concentrated than thyroxine
D) Concentrations of chloride and thyroxine are equal
E) Thyroxine is 1000 times more concentrated than chloride
F) Thyroxine is 1,000,000 times more concentrated than chloride

Question 32:
Which of the following is **NOT** a hormone?

A) Insulin
B) Glycogen
C) Noradrenaline
D) Cortisol
E) Thyroxine
F) Progesterone
G) None of the above

Question 33:
Which of the following statements regarding neural reflexes is **FALSE**?

A) Reflexes are usually faster than voluntary decisions
B) Reflex actions are faster than endocrine responses
C) The heat-withdrawal reflex is an example of a spinal reflex
D) Reflexes are completely unaffected by the brain
E) Reflexes are present in simple animals
F) Reflexes have both a sensory and motor component

Question 34:
The table below shows the results of a study investigating antibiotic resistance in staphylococcus populations.

Antibiotic	Number of Bacteria tested	Number of Resistant Bacteria
Benzyl-penicillin	10^{11}	98
Chloramphenicol	10^{9}	1200
Metronidazole	10^{8}	256
Erythtomycin	10^{5}	2

A single staphylococcus bacterium is chosen at random from a similar population. Resistance to any one antibiotic is independent of resistance to others.

Calculate the probability that the bacterium selected will be resistant to all four drugs.
A) 1 in 10^{12} B) 1 in 10^{6} C) 1 in 10^{20} D) 1 in 10^{25} E) 1 in 10^{30} F) 1 in 10^{35}

Question 35:
Which of the following components of a food chain represent the largest biomass?

A) Producers
B) Decomposers
C) Primary consumers
D) Secondary consumers
E) Tertiary consumers

Question 36:
Why does air flow into the chest on inspiration?

1. Atmospheric pressure is smaller than intra-thoracic pressure during inspiration.
2. Atmospheric pressure is greater than intra-thoracic pressure during inspiration.
3. Anterior and lateral chest expansion decreases absolute intra-thoracic pressure.
4. Anterior and lateral chest expansion increases absolute intra-thoracic pressure.

A) 1 only
B) 2 only
C) 2 and 3
D) 1 and 4
E) 1 and 3
F) 2 and 4

Question 37:
Concerning the nitrogen cycle, which of the following are true?

1. The majority of the Earth's atmosphere is nitrogen.
2. Most of the nitrogen in the Earth's atmosphere is inert.
3. Bacteria are essential for nitrogen fixation.
4. Nitrogen fixation occurs during lightning strikes.

A) 1 and 2
B) 1 and 3
C) 2 and 3
D) 2 and 4
E) 3 and 4
F) 1, 2, 3 and 4

Question 38:
Which of the following statement are correct regarding mutations?

1. Mutations always cause proteins to lose their function.
2. Mutations always change the structure of the protein encoded by the affected gene.
3. Mutations always result in cancer.

A) Only 1
B) Only 2
C) Only 3
D) 1 and 2
E) 2 and 3
F) 1 and 3
G) 1, 2 and 3
H) None of the above

Question 39:
Which of the following is not a function of the central nervous system?

A) Coordination of movement
B) Decision making and executive functions
C) Control of heart rate
D) Cognition
E) Memory

Question 40:
Which of the following control mechanisms are involved in modulating cardiac output?

1. Voluntary control.
2. Sympathetic control to decrease heart rate.
3. Parasympathetic control to increase heart rate.

A) Only 1
B) Only 2
C) Only 3
D) 1 and 2
E) 2 and 3
F) 1 and 3
G) 1, 2 and 3
H) None of the above

END OF SECTION

Section 3

Question 41:
Place the following substances in order from most to least reactive:

1. Sodium
2. Potassium
3. Aluminium
4. Zinc
5. Copper
6. Magnesium

A) 1 » 2 » 6 » 3 » 4 » 5
B) 1 » 2 » 6 » 3 » 5 » 4
C) 2 » 1 » 6 » 3 » 4 » 5
D) 2 » 1 » 6 » 3 » 5 » 4
E) 2 » 6 » 1 » 3 » 4 » 5

Question 42:
A cup has 144ml of pure deionised water. How many electrons are in the cup due to the water? [Avogadro Constant = 6×10^{23}]

A) 8.64×10^{24}
B) 8.64×10^{25}
C) 1.2×10^{24}
D) 4.8×10^{24}
E) 4.8×10^{25}

Question 43:
Steve's sports car requires 2.28kg of octane to travel to Pete's house 10 miles away. Calculate the mass of CO_2 produced during the journey.

A) 0.88 kg
B) 1.66 kg
C) 2.64 kg
D) 3.52 kg
E) 5.28 kg
F) 7.04 kg

Question 44:
In which of the following mixtures will a displacement reaction occur?

1. $Cu + 2AgNO_3$
2. $Cu + Fe(NO_3)_2$
3. $Ca + 2H_2O$
4. $Fe + Ca(OH)_2$

A) 1 only
B) 2 only
C) 3 only
D) 4 only
E) 1 and 2 only
F) 1 and 3 only
G) 1, 2 and 3
H) 1, 2, 3 and 4

Question 45:
Which of the following statements is true about the following chain of metals?

$Na \rightarrow Ca \rightarrow Mg \rightarrow Al \rightarrow Zn$
Moving from left to right:

1. The reactivity of the metals increases.
2. The likelihood of corrosion of the metals increases.
3. More energy is required to separate these metals from their ores.
4. The metals lose electrons more readily to form positive ions.

A) 1 and 2 only
B) 1 and 3 only
C) 2 and 3 only
D) 1 and 4 only
E) 2, 3 and 4 only
F) 1, 2, 3 and 4
G) None of the above

Question 46:
In which of the following mixtures will a displacement reaction occur?

1. $I_2 + 2KBr$
2. $Cl_2 + 2NaBr$
3. $Br_2 + 2KI$

A) 1 only
B) 2 only
C) 3 only
D) 1 and 2 only
E) 1 and 3 only
F) 2 and 3 only
G) 1, 2 and 3

Question 47:
Which of the following statements about Al and Cu are true?

1. Al is used to build aircraft because it is lightweight and resists corrosion.
2. Cu is used to build electrical wires because it is a good insulator.
3. Both Al and Cu are good conductors of heat.
4. Al is commonly alloyed with other metals to make coins.
5. Al is resistant to corrosion because of a thin layer of aluminium hydroxide on its surface.

A) 1 and 3 only
B) 1 and 4 only
C) 1, 3 and 5 only
D) 1, 3, 4, 5 only
E) 2, 4 and 5 only
F) 2, 3, 4, 5 only

Question 48:
21g of Li^7 reacts completely with excess water. Given that the molar gas volume is 24 dm^3 under the conditions, what is the volume of hydrogen produced?

A) 12 dm^3
B) 24 dm^3
C) 36 dm^3
D) 48 dm^3
E) 72 dm^3
F) 120 dm^3

Question 49:
Which of the following statements regarding bonding are true?

1. NaCl has stronger ionic bonds than $MgCl_2$
2. Transition metals are able to lose varying numbers of electrons to form multiple stable positive ions.
3. All covalently bonded structures have lower melting points than ionically bonded compounds.
4. All covalently bonded structures do not conduct electricity.

A) 1 only
B) 2 only
C) 3 only
D) 4 only
E) 1 and 2 only
F) 2 and 3 only
G) 3 and 4 only
H) 1, 2 and 4 only

Question 50:
Which of the following pairs have the same electronic configuration?

1. Li^+ and Na^+
2. Mg^{2+} and Ne
3. Na^{2+} and Ne
4. O^{2-} and a Carbon atom

A) 1 only
B) 1 and 2 only
C) 1 and 3 only
D) 2 and 3 only
E) 2 and 4 only
F) 1, 2, 3 and 4

Question 51:
Consider the following two equations:

A.	$C + O_2 \rightarrow CO_2$	$\Delta H = -394$ kJ per mole
B.	$CaCO_3 \rightarrow CaO + CO_2$	$\Delta H = +178$ kJ per mole

Which of the following statements are true?

1. Reaction A is exothermic and Reaction B is endothermic
2. CO_2 has less energy than C and O_2.
3. CaO is more stable than $CaCO_3$.

A) 1 only
B) 2 only
C) 3 only
D) 1 and 2
E) 1 and 3
F) 2 and 3
G) 1, 2 and 3

Question 52:
Which of the following are true of regarding the oxides formed by Na, Mg and Al?

1. All of the metals and their solid oxides conduct electricity.
2. MgO has stronger bonds than Na_2O.
3. Metals are extracted from their molten ores by fractional distillation.

A) 1 only
B) 2 only
C) 3 only
D) 1 and 2 only
E) 2 and 3 only
F) 1, 2 and 3

END OF SECTION

Section 4

Question 53:

Calculate the radius of a sphere which has a surface area three times as great as its volume.

A) 0.5
B) 1
C) 1.5
D) 2
E) 2.5
F) More information is needed

Question 54:

A mechanical winch lifts up a bag of grain in a mill from the floor into a hopper.

Assuming that the machine is 100% efficient and lifts the bag vertically only, which of the following statements are **TRUE**?

1. This increases gravitational potential energy
2. The gravitational potential energy is independent of the mass of the grain
3. The work done is the difference between the gravitational potential energy at the hopper and when the grain is on the floor
4. The work done is the difference between the kinetic energy of the grain in the hopper and on the floor

A) 1 only
B) 1 and 3
C) 1 and 4
D) 1, 2 and 3
E) 1, 2 and 4
F) None of the above

Question 55:

A barometer records atmospheric pressure as 10^5 Pa. Recalling that the diameter of the Earth is 1.2×10^7 m, **estimate** the mass of the atmosphere. [Assume $g = 10\ ms^{-2}$, the earth is spherical and that $\pi=3$]

A) 4.5×10^8 kg
B) 4.5×10^{10} kg
C) 4.5×10^{12} kg
D) 4.5×10^{13} kg
E) 4.5×10^{18} kg
F) More information is required

Question 56:

A 6kg missile is fired and decelerates at $6ms^{-2}$.

What is the difference in resistive force compared to a 2kg missile fired and decelerating at $8ms^{-2}$?

A) 8N
B) 12N
C) 16N
D) 20N
E) 24N

Question 57:

There are 1000 international airports in the world. If 4 flights take off every hour from each airport, estimate the annual number of commercial flights worldwide, to the nearest 1 million.

A) 20 million
B) 35 million
C) 37 million
D) 40 million
E) 42 million
F) 44 million

Question 58:

The figure below shows a schematic of a wiring system. All the bulbs have equal resistance. The power supply is 24V.

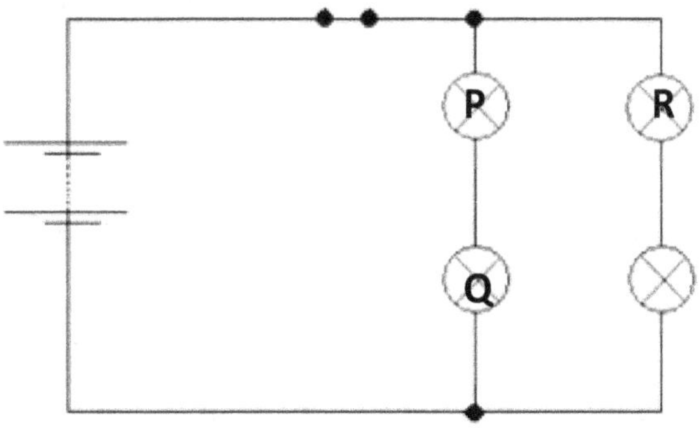

If headlight Q is replaced by a new one with twice the resistance, with the switch closed, which of these combinations of voltage drop across the four bulbs is possible?

	P	Q	R	S
A)	8V	16V	12V	12V
B)	8V	16V	16V	8V
C)	8V	16V	8V	16V
D)	12V	24V	24V	24V
E)	12V	12V	12V	12V
F)	16V	8V	12V	12V
G)	16V	8V	8V	16V
H)	24V	24V	24V	24V
I)	4V	8V	6V	6V
J)	8V	4V	6V	6V

Question 59:

Given:

$F + G + H = 1$

$F + G - H = 2$

$F - G - H = 3$

Calculate the value of FGH.

A) -2　　B) -0.5　　C) 0　　D) 0.5　　E) 2

Question 60:
Put the following types of electromagnetic waves in ascending order of wavelength:

	Shortest -			- Longest
A)	Visible Light	Ultraviolet	Infrared	X Ray
B)	Visible Light	Infrared	Ultraviolet	X Ray
C)	Infrared	Visible Light	Ultraviolet	X Ray
D)	Infrared	Visible Light	X Ray	Ultraviolet
E)	X Ray	Ultraviolet	Visible Light	Infrared
F)	X Ray	Ultraviolet	Infrared	Visible Light
G)	Ultraviolet	X Ray	Visible Light	Infrared

END OF PAPER

MOCK PAPER E

Section 1

Question 1:
"Peter books a return flight to Dubai for £725. The flight is refundable, but there is a fee of £45 payable for cancelling. Peter notices as time passes, the remaining tickets on the same plane are becoming cheaper. He decides to cancel his flight, booking a new one for £530 through the same provider. Once again he sees prices have fallen, so he cancels this flight but can only buy a new one for £495."

What is his overall saving, relative to the original price paid?

A) £110 B) £140 C) £150 D) £195 E) £230

Question 2:
"You have three bags, each containing four balls numbered with single digit numbers. Bag A contains even numbers only, Bag B contains odd numbers only, and Bag C contains the numbers 2, 5, 6 and 8. You take a ball from Bag B and put it into Bag C; then you then take a ball from Bag C and put it into Bag A. You draw a ball at random from Bag A."

What is the probability that this ball is an odd number?

A) $^1/_{25}$ B) $^2/_{25}$ C) $^3/_{25}$ D) $^4/_{25}$ E) $^1/_5$

Question 3:
The price of bread rises by 40% due to a poor grain harvest. This is later reduced by 20% due to a government farming subsidy. Dave buys three loaves of bread and gets a fourth free because of a discount in the shop.

How much did he pay per loaf of bread? Express your answer as a percentage of the original price.

A) 66% B) 84% C) 92% D) 98% E) 110%

Question 4:
Sam notes that the time on a normal analogue clock is 2120hrs. What is the smaller angle between the hands on the clock?

A) 130° B) 140° C) 150° D) 160° E) 170°

Question 5:
Sam needs to measure out exactly 4 litres of water into a tank. He has two pieces of equipment – a bucket that holds 5 litres and a one that holds 3 litres, with no intermediate markings.

Is it possible to measure out 4 litres? If so, how much water is needed in total in order to measure the 4 litres?

A) 4 litres
B) 7 litres
C) 8 litres
D) 10 litres
E) Not possible with this equipment

Question 6:

"A librarian is sorting books into their correct locations. All history books belong to the right of all science books. Science books are divided into five locations: engineering, biology, chemistry, physics and mathematics (in an uninterrupted order from right to left). Art books are located to the right of mathematics between engineering and sport, and sport books between art and history. Literature books are to the right of art books."

What can be certainly said about the location of literature books?

A) They are located between art and history books
B) They are located to the left of history books
C) They are located between mathematics and art
D) They are located to the right of engineering
E) They are not located to the left of sport

Question 7:

"Many people choose not to buy brand new cars, as buying brand new has significant disadvantages. Most importantly, a car's value drops substantially the moment it is first driven on the road. Even though a car is virtually unchanged by these first few miles, the potential resale value is significantly reduced. Therefore it is better to buy second hand cars, as their value does not drop so much immediately after purchase."

Which of the following best represents the main conclusion of this passage?

A) There are many equal reasons to avoid buying brand new cars
B) Cars that have driven lots of miles should be avoided
C) The rapid loss of value of new cars makes buying second-hand a wise choice
D) Second hand cars are at least as good as new ones
E) New cars should not be driven to ensure they keep their resale value

Question 8:

James is a wine dealer specialising in French wine. From his original stock of 2,000 bottles in one cellar, he sells 10% to one customer and 20% of the remaining wine to another customer. He makes £11,200 profit from the two transactions combined. What is the average profit per bottle?

A) £18 B) £20 C) £22 D) £24 E) £26

Question 9:

"Many good quality pieces of old furniture are considered 'timeless' – they are used and enjoyed by many people today, and this is expected to continue for many generations to come. However, most of this furniture dates back to previous eras, and modern furniture does not fall under the 'timeless' category of being enjoyed for many years to come."

Which of the following is the main flaw in the argument?
A) There may be many factors which make furniture good
B) There used to be more furniture makers than today
C) No evidence is given to tell us old furniture is better than new
D) Old furniture is desirable for other reasons than its quality
E) We cannot yet tell whether new furniture will become 'timeless'

Question 10:
"Red wine is thought to be much healthier than beer because it contains many antioxidants, which have been shown to be beneficial to health. Many red wines are produced in Southern France and Italy, therefore it is no surprise that residents there have a greater life expectancy than in the UK and Germany, which are predominantly beer producing countries."

Which of the following is an assumption of the above argument?

A) Italian people drink red wine
B) Antioxidants are beneficial for health
C) British people prefer beer to red wine
D) Beer is not produced in Italy
E) Italian life expectancy is greater than in the UK

Question 11:
Hannah, Jane and Tom are travelling to London to see a musical. Hannah catches the train at 1430. Jane leaves at the same time as Hannah, but catches a bus which takes 40% longer then Hannah's train. Tom also takes a train, and the journey time is 10 minutes less then Hannah's journey, but he leaves 45 minutes after Jane leaves. He arrives in London at 1620.

At what time will Jane arrive in London?

A) 1545 B) 1600 C) 1615 D) 1700 E) 1715

Question 12:
At a show, there are two different ticket prices for different seats. The cost is £10 for a standard seat, and £16 for a premium view seat. The total revenue from a show is £6,600, and the total attendance was 600.

How many premium view seats were purchased?

A) 60 B) 100 C) 140 D) 180 E) 240

Question 13:
The moon orbits the Earth once every 28 days. Between 20th January and 23rd May inclusive, how many degrees has the Moon turned through? This is not a leap year.

A) 1540° B) 1560° C) 1580° D) 1600° E) 1620°

Question 14:
Drama academies are special schools students can go to in order to learn performing arts. These schools are only available to the most skilled young performers, and aim to give students the best training in the arts, whilst still covering mainstream academic subjects. However, many parents are reluctant for their children to attend such academies, as they feel the academic teaching will be worse than at a standard school.

Which of the following, if true, would most weaken the above argument?

A) Most top actors attended a drama academy as children
B) There is as much time dedicated to academic work in drama academies as there is in normal schools
C) The academic work comprises a greater proportion of the study time than drama related activities
D) Most children are keen to attend a drama academy if given the opportunity
E) 80% of students at drama academies attain higher than average GCSE scores

Question 15:

Anil and Suresh both leave point A at the same time. Anil travels 5km East then 10km North. Anil then travels a further 1km North before heading 3km West. Suresh travels East for 2km less than Anil's total journey distance. He then heads 13km North, before pausing and travelling back 2km South. How far, as the crow flies, are the two men now apart?

A) 11km B) 12km C) 13km D) 15km E) 17km

Question 16:

Chris leaves his house to go and visit Laura, who lives 3 miles away. He leaves at 1730 and walks at 4mph towards Laura's house, stopping for one 5-minute to chat to a friend. Meanwhile Sarah also wants to visit Laura. She sets off from her house 6 miles away at 1810, driving in her car and averaging a speed of 24mph.

Who reaches the house first and with how long do they wait for the other person?

A) Chris, and waits 5 mins for Sarah
B) Chris, and waits 10 mins for Sarah
C) Sarah, and waits 5 mins for Chris
D) Sarah, and waits 10 mins for Chris
E) They both arrive at the same time

Question 17:

"Illegal film and music downloads have increased greatly in recent years. This causes significant harm to the relevant industries. Many people justify this to themselves by telling themselves they are only diverting money away from wealthy and successful singers and actors, who do not need any more money anyway. But in reality, illegal downloads are deeply harming the music industry, making many studio workers redundant and making it difficult for less famous performers to make a living."

Which of the following best summarises the conclusion of this argument?

A) Unemployment is a problem in the music industry
B) Taking profits away from successful musicians does more harm than good
C) Studio workers are most affected by illegal downloads
D) Illegal downloads cause more harm than people often think
E) Buying music legally helps keep the music industry productive

Question 18:

"40,000 litres of water will extinguish two typical house fires. 70,000 litres of water will extinguish two house fires and three garden fires. There is no surplus water"

Which statement is **NOT** true?

A) A garden fire can be extinguished with 12,000 litres, with water to spare.
B) 20,000 litres is sufficient to extinguish a normal house fire.
C) A garden fire requires only half as much water to extinguish as a house fire.
D) Two house and four garden fires will need 80,000 litres to extinguish.
E) Three house and ten garden fires will need 140,000 litres to extinguish.

Question 19:
"Plans are in place to install antennas underground, so that users of underground trains will be able to pick up mobile reception. There are, as usual, winners and losers from this policy. Supporters of the policy argue that it will lead to an increase in workforce productivity and increase convenience in day-to-day life. Critics respond by saying that it will lead to an annoying environment whilst travelling, it will facilitate the ease of conducting a terrorist threat and it will decrease levels of sociability. The latter camp seems to have the greatest support and so a re-consideration of the policy is urged."

Which of the following **best** summarises the conclusion of this passage?

A) The disadvantages of installing underground antennas outweigh the benefits
B) The cost of the scheme is likely to be prohibitive
C) The policy must be dropped, since a majority does not want it
D) More people don't want this scheme than do want it
E) A detailed consultation process should take place

Question 20:
"Ecosystems in the oceans are changing. Recently, restrictions on fishing have been imposed to tackle the decline in fish populations. As a result, farm fishing and the price of fish have increased, whilst the seas recover. It is hoped that these changes will lead to a brighter future for all."

Which of the following are **TWO** assumptions of this argument?

A) People will still buy farmed fish at a higher price
B) The population of wild fish can recover
C) Fishermen will benefit from working on this scheme
D) Ecosystems have been altered as a result of climate change
E) Heavy sea fishing is to blame for the changes in the ecosystem

Question 21:
Who wrote *Ullyses?*

A) Homer
B) Plato
C) Virginia Wollf
D) James Joyce
E) Marcel Proust

Question 22:
Who succeeded Ban Ki-Moon as Secretary-General of the UN in 2017?

A) Tony Blair
B) Bill Clinton
C) Kofi Annan
D) Barack Obama
E) Antonio Guterres

END OF SECTION

Section 2

Question 23:
Which of the following statements, regarding normal human digestion, is **FALSE**?

A) Amylase is an enzyme which breaks down starch
B) Amylase is produced by the pancreas
C) Bile is stored in the gallbladder
D) The small intestine is the longest part of the gut
E) Insulin is released in response to feeding
F) None of the above

Question 24:
Jane is one mile into a marathon. Which of the following statements is **NOT** true, relative to before she started?

A) Blood flow to the skin is increased
B) Blood flow to the muscles is increased
C) Blood flow to the gut is decreased
D) Blood flow to the kidneys is decreased
E) Cardiac Output Increases
F) None of the above

Question 25:
A newly discovered species of beetle is found to have 29.6% Adenine (A) bases in its genome. What is the percentage of Cytosine (C) bases in the beetle's DNA?

A) 20.4%
B) 29.6%
C) 40.8%
D) 59.2%
E) 70.6%
F) More information is required

Question 26:
Carbon monoxide binds irreversibly to the oxygen binding site of haemoglobin. Which of the following statements is true regarding carbon monoxide poisoning?

A) Carbon monoxide poisoning has no serious consequences
B) Haemoglobin is heavier, as both oxygen and carbon monoxide bind to it
C) Affected individuals have a raised heart rate
D) The CO_2 carrying capacity of the blood is decreased
E) The O_2 carrying capacity of the blood is unchanged as it dissolves in the plasma instead

Question 27:
Antibiotics can have serious side effects such as liver failure and renal failure. Therefore, scientists are always trying to develop antibiotics to minimise these effects by targeting specific cellular components. Which of these cellular components offers the best way to treat infections and minimise side effects?

A) Mitochondrion
B) Cell membrane
C) Nucleic acid
D) Cytoskeleton
E) Flagellum

Question 28:
Study the following diagram of the human heart. What is true about structure **A**?

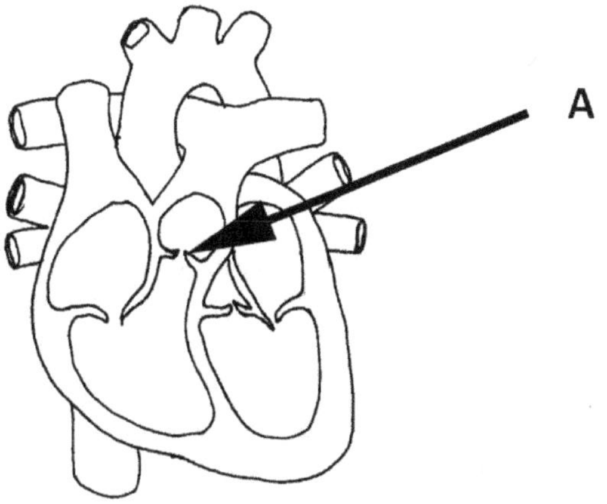

A) It is closed during systole
B) It prevents blood flowing into the left ventricle during systole
C) It prevents blood flowing into the right ventricle during systole
D) It prevents blood flowing into the left ventricle during diastole
E) It opens due to left ventricular pressure being greater than aortic pressure.
F) It is open when the right ventricle is emptying

Question 29:
A person responds to the starting gun of a race and begins to run. Place the following order of events in the most likely chronological sequence. Which option is a correct sequence?

1 Blood CO_2 increases
2 The eardrum vibrates to the sound
3 Impulses travel along motor neurones
4 Impulses travel along sensory neurones
5 Impulses travel along relay neurones
6 Quadriceps muscles contract
7 Glycogen is converted into glucose
8 Creatine phosphate rapidly re-phosphorylates ADP

A) $2 \rightarrow 5 \rightarrow 4 \rightarrow 3 \rightarrow 6 \rightarrow 7$
B) $2 \rightarrow 4 \rightarrow 3 \rightarrow 8 \rightarrow 6 \rightarrow 1$
C) $2 \rightarrow 3 \rightarrow 4 \rightarrow 6 \rightarrow 7 \rightarrow 1$
D) $2 \rightarrow 4 \rightarrow 3 \rightarrow 1 \rightarrow 6 \rightarrow 7$
E) $2 \rightarrow 4 \rightarrow 3 \rightarrow 6 \rightarrow 8 \rightarrow 7$

Question 30:
Which of the following best describes the events that occur during expiration?

A) The ribs move up and in; the diaphragm moves down.
B) The ribs move down and in; the diaphragm moves up.
C) The ribs move up and in; the diaphragm moves up.
D) The ribs move down and out; the diaphragm moves down.
E) The ribs move up and out; the diaphragm moves down.
F) The ribs move up and out; the diaphragm moves up.

Question 31:
Vijay goes to see his GP with fatty, smelly stools that float on water. Which of the following enzymes is most likely to be malfunctioning?

A) Amylase
B) Lipase
C) Protease
D) Sucrase
E) Lactase
F)

Question 32:
Which of the following statements concerning the cardiovascular system is correct?

A) Oxygenated blood from the lungs flows to the heart via the pulmonary artery.
B) All arteries carry oxygenated blood.
C) All animals have a double circulatory system.
D) The superior vena cava contains oxygenated blood
E) All veins have valves.
F) None of the above.

Question 33:
Which part of the GI tract has the least amount of enzymatic digestion occurring?

A) Mouth
B) Stomach
C) Small intestine
D) Large intestine
E) Rectum

Question 34:
Oge touches a hot stove and immediately moves her hand away. Which of the following components are **NOT** involved in this reaction?

1. Thermo-receptor
2. Brain
3. Spinal Cord
4. Sensory nerve
5. Motor nerve
6. Muscle

A) 1 only
B) 2 only
C) 3 only
D) 1 and 2 only
E) 1, 2 and 3 only
F) 3, 4, 5 and 6

Question 35:
Which of the following represents a scenario with an appropriate description of the mode of transport?

1. Water moving from a hypotonic solution outside of a potato cell, across the cell wall and cell membrane and into the hypertonic cytoplasm of the potato cell→ Osmosis.
2. Carbon dioxide moving across a respiring cell's membrane and dissolving in blood plasma →Active transport.
3. Reabsorption of amino acids against a concentration gradient in the glomeruluar apparatus → Diffusion.

A) 1 only
B) 2 only
C) 3 only
D) 1 and 2 only
E) 2 and 3 only
F) 1 and 3 only
G) 1, 2 and 3

Question 36:
Which of the following equations represents anaerobic respiration?

1. Carbohydrate + Oxygen → Energy + Carbon Dioxide + Water
2. Carbohydrate → Energy + Lactic Acid + Carbon dioxide
3. Carbohydrate → Energy + Lactic Acid
4. Carbohydrate → Energy + Ethanol + Carbon dioxide

A) 1 only
B) 2 only
C) 3 only
D) 4 only
E) 1 and 2
F) 1 and 3
G) 1 and 4
H) 2 and 4 only
I) 3 and 4 only

Question 37:
Which of the following statements regarding respiration are correct?

1. The mitochondria are the centres for both aerobic and anaerobic respiration.
2. The cytoplasm is the main site of anaerobic respiration.
3. For every two moles of glucose that is respired aerobically, 12 moles of CO_2 are liberated.
4. Anaerobic respiration is more efficient than aerobic respiration.

A) 1 and 2
B) 1 and 4
C) 2 and 3
D) 2 and 4
E) 3 and 4

Question 38:
Which of the following statements are true?

1. The nucleus contains the cell's chromosomes.
2. The cytoplasm consists purely of water.
3. The plasma membrane is a single phospholipid layer.
4. The cell wall prevents plants cells from lysing due to osmotic pressure.

A) 1 and 2
B) 1 and 4
C) 1, 3 and 4
D) 1, 2 and 3
E) 1, 2 and 4
F) 2, 3 and 4

Question 39:

Which of the following statements are true about osmosis?

1. If a medium is hypertonic relative to the cell cytoplasm, the cell will gain water through osmosis.
2. If a medium is hypotonic relative to the cell cytoplasm, the cell will gain water through osmosis.
3. If a medium is hypotonic relative to the cell cytoplasm, the cell will lose water through osmosis.
4. If a medium is hypertonic relative to the cell cytoplasm, the cell will lose water through osmosis.
5. The medium's tonicity has no impact on the movement of water.

A) 1 only
B) 2 only
C) 1 and 3
D) 2 and 4
E) 5 only

Question 40:
Which of the following statements are true about stem cells?

1. Stem cells have the ability to differentiate into other mature types of cells.
2. Stem cells are unable to maintain their undifferentiated state.
3. Stem cells can be classified as embryonic stem cells or adult stem cells.
4. Stem cells are only found in embryos.

A) 1 and 3
B) 3 and 4
C) 2 and 3
D) 1 and 2
E) 2 and 4

END OF SECTION

Section 3

Question 41:
Which of the following below is **NOT** an example of an oxidation reaction?

A) $Li^{+} + H_2O \rightarrow Li^{+} + OH^{-} + \frac{1}{2}H_2$
B) $N_2 \rightarrow 2N^{+} + 2e^{-}$
C) $2CH_4 + 2O_2 \rightarrow 2CH_2O + 2H_2O$
D) $2N_2 + O_2 \rightarrow 2N_2O$
E) $I_2 + 2e^{-} \rightarrow 2I^{-}$
F) All of the above are oxidation reactions

Question 42:
Balance the following chemical equation. What is the value of **x**?

w $HIO_3 + 4FeI_2 +$ **x** $HCl \rightarrow$ **y** $FeCl_3 +$ **z** $ICl + 15H_2O$

A) 4
B) 5
C) 9
D) 15
E) 22
F) 25

Question 43:
On analysis, an organic substance is found to contain 41.4% Carbon, 55.2% Oxygen and 3.45% Hydrogen by mass. Which of the following could be the chemical formula of this substance?

A) $C_3O_3H_6$
B) $C_3O_3H_{12}$
C) $C_4O_2H_4$
D) $C_4O_4H_4$
E) $C_4O_2H_8$
F) More information needed

Question 44:
200 cm^3 of a 1.8 moldm^{-3} solution of sodium nitrate ($NaNO_3$) is used in a chemical reaction. How many moles of sodium nitrate is this?

A) 0.09 mol
B) 0.36 mol
C) 9.00 mol
D) 36.0 mol
E) 360 mol

Question 45:
A is a group 3 element and B is a group 6 element. Which row best describes what happens to A when it reacts with B?

	Electrons are	Size of Atom
A)	Gained	Increases
B)	Gained	Decreases
C)	Gained	Unchanged
D)	Lost	Increases
E)	Lost	Decreases
F)	Lost	Unchanged

Question 46:
In relation to reactivity of elements in group 1 and 2, which of the following statements is correct?

1. Reactivity decreases as you go down group 1.
2. Reactivity increases as you go down group 2.
3. Group 1 metals are generally less reactive than group 2 metals.

A) Only 1
B) Only 2
C) Only 3
D) 1 and 2
E) 2 and 3
F) 1 and 3

Question 47:
What role do catalysts fulfil in an endothermic reaction?

A) They increase the temperature, causing the reaction to occur at a faster rate.
B) They decrease the temperature, causing the reaction to occur at a faster rate.
C) They reduce the energy of the reactants in order to trigger the reaction.
D) They reduce the activation energy of the reaction.
E) They increase the activation energy of the reaction.

Question 48:
Tritium H^3 is an isotope of Hydrogen. Why is tritium commonly referred to as 'heavy hydrogen'?

A) Because H^3 contains 3 protons making it heavier than H^1 that contains 1 proton.
B) Because H^3 contains 3 neutrons making it heavier than H^1 that contains 1 neutron.
C) Because H^3 contains 1 neutron and 2 protons making it heavier than H^1 that contains 1 neutron and 1 proton.
D) Because H^3 contains 1 proton and 2 neutrons making it heavier than H^1 that contains 1 proton.
E) Because H^3 contains 3 electrons making it heavier than H^1 that contains 1 electron.

Question 49:
Which of the following statements is correct?

A) At higher temperatures, gas molecules move at angles that cause them to collide with each other more frequently.
B) Gas molecules have lower energy after colliding with each other.
C) At higher temperatures, gas molecules attract each other resulting in more collisions.
D) The average kinetic energy of gas molecules is the same for all gases at the same temperature.
E) The momentum of gas molecules decreases as pressure increases.

Question 50:
In relation to redox reactions, which of the following statements are correct?

1. Oxidation describes the loss of electrons.
2. Reduction increases the electron density of an ion, atom or molecule.
3. Halogens are powerful reducing agents.

A) Only 1
B) Only 2
C) Only 3
D) 1 and 2
E) 2 and 3
F) 1 and 3

Question 51:
Which of the following are exothermic reactions?

1. Burning Magnesium in pure oxygen
2. The combustion of hydrogen
3. Aerobic respiration
4. Evaporation of water in the oceans
5. Reaction between a strong acid and a strong base

A) 1, 2 and 4
B) 1, 2 and 5
C) 1, 3 and 5
D) 2, 3 and 4
E) 1, 2, 3 and 5
F) 1, 2, 3, 4 and 5

Question 52:
Ethene reacts with oxygen to produce water and carbon dioxide. Which elements are oxidised/reduced?

A) Carbon is reduced, and oxygen is oxidised.
B) Hydrogen is reduced, and oxygen is oxidised.
C) Carbon is oxidised, and hydrogen is reduced.
D) Hydrogen is oxidised, and carbon is reduced.
E) Carbon is oxidised, and oxygen is reduced.
F) None of the above.

END OF SECTION

Section 4

Question 53:
The buoyancy force of an object is the produce of its volume, density and the gravitational constant, *g*. A boat weighing 600 kg with a density of 1000kgm^{-3} and hull volume of 950 litres is placed in a lake. What is the minimum mass that, if added to the boat, will cause it to sink? Use g = 10ms^{-1}.

A) 3.55 kg B) 35 kg C) 350 kg D) 355 kg E) 3550 kg F) None

Question 54:
Mr Khan fires a bullet at a speed of 310 ms^{-1} from a height of 1.93m parallel to the floor. Mr Weeks drops an identical bullet from the same height.

What is the time difference between the bullets first making contact with the floor?[Assume that there is negligible air resistance; *g*= 10 ms^{-2}]

A) 0 s
B) 0.2 s
C) 1.93 s
D) 2.1 s
E) More information needed

Question 55:
A 1.4kg fish swims through water at a constant speed of 2ms^{-1}. Resistive forces against the fish are 2N. Assuming g = 10ms^{-2}, how much work does the fish do in one hour?

A) 7,200 J
B) 10,080 J
C) 14,400 J
D) 19,880 J
E) 22,500 J
F) More information needed

Question 56:
A crane is 40 m tall. The lifting arm is 5m long and the counterbalance arm is 2m long. The beam joining the two weighs 350kg, and is of uniform thickness. The lifting arm lifts a 2000 kg mass. What counterbalance mass is required to balance exactly around the centre point? Use g = 10 ms^{-2}.

A) 4,220 kg
B) 4,820 kg
C) 5,013 kg
D) 5,263 kg
E) 10,525 kg

Question 57:
For Christmas, Mr James decorates his house with 20 strings of 150 bulbs each. Each 150-bulb string of lights is rated at 50 Watts. Mr James turns the lights on at 8pm and off at 6am each night. The lights are used for 20 days in total.

If 100 kJ of energy costs 2p, how much is the total cost Mr James has to pay?

A) £2160.00 B) £144.00 C) £14.40 D) £0.72 E) £0.24

Question 58:
Calculate the perimeter of a regular polygon each interior angle is 150° and each side is 15 cm.

A) 75 cm
B) 150 cm
C) 180 cm
D) 225 cm
E) 1,500 cm
F) More information needed.

Question 59:
The diagram shown below depicts an electrical circuit with multiple resistors, each with equal resistance, *Z*. The total resistance between A and B is 22 MΩ. Calculate the value of *Z*.

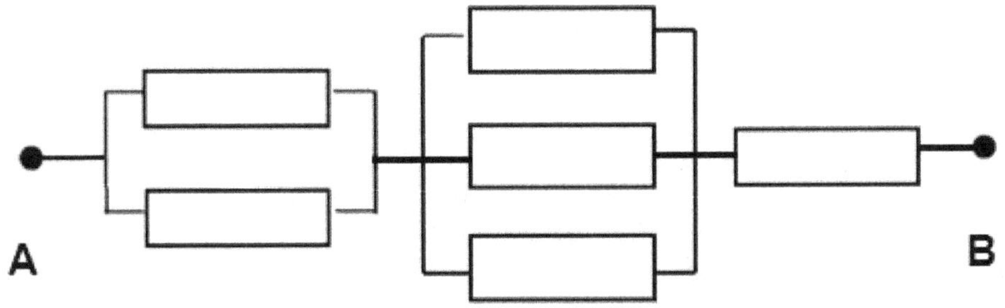

A) 3.33 MΩ B) 4.33 MΩ C) 7.33 MΩ D) 11 MΩ E) 12 MΩ

Question 60:
A cylindrical candle of diameter 4cm burns steadily at a rate of 1cm per hour. Assuming the candle is composed entirely of paraffin wax ($C_{24}H_{52}$) of density 900 kgm^{-3} and undergoes complete combustion, how much energy is transferred in 30 minutes? You may assume the molar combustion energy is 11,000 $kJmol^{-1}$, and that π=3.

A) 140,000J
B) 175,000J
C) 185,000J
D) 200,500J
E) 215,000J
F) 348,000J

END OF PAPER

MOCK PAPER F

Section 1

Question 1:
Every year, there are tens of thousands of motor crashes, causing a serious number of fatalities. Indeed, this represents the leading cause of death in the UK that is not a disease. In spite of this horrendous statistic, there are still thousands of uninsured drivers. The government is under moral obligation to clamp down on uninsured drivers, to reduce the incidence of such crashes. That they have not acted is arguably the most outrageous failing of the present government.

Which of the following is the best statement of a **flaw** in this passage?

A) It has made unsupported claims that the government's failure to act is morally outrageous.
B) It has not provided any evidence to support its claims that motor crashes are the leading cause of death in the UK outside of diseases.
C) Even if motor crashes were prevented, it would not save lives of people who die from other causes.
D) It has implied that lack of insurance is related to the incidence of motor crashes.
E) It has fabricated an obligation on the government's part to intervene and reduce the numbers of uninsured drivers.

Question 2:
Several years ago the Brazilian government held a referendum of the populace, to decide whether they should enact a law banning the ownership of guns. The Brazilian people voted strongly against this proposal. When asked why this had happened, one commentator said he believed the reason was that 90% of criminals who use guns to commit crimes buy their weapons on the black market, illegally. Thus, if Brazil were to ban the legal sale of guns, this would remove the ability of law-abiding citizens to purchase protection, whilst doing little to remove weapons from the hands of criminals.

Some commentators have pointed to this statistic, and claimed that the UK should also legalise guns, to allow citizens to protect themselves. However, in the UK the black market for weapons is not as widespread as in Brazil. Most people in the UK have little reason to fear gun attacks, and legalising the sale of guns would simply make it much easier for criminals to acquire weapons.

Which of the following best expresses the main conclusion of this passage?

A) The UK should not follow Brazil's lead on gun legislation.
B) Efforts to reduce gun ownership should focus on the black market.
C) Violent crime is a more pressing concern in Brazil than the UK.
D) Legalising the sale of guns in the UK would result in widespread ownership.
E) Criminals will always find a way to obtain firearms.

Question 3:
Hannah is buying tiles for her new bathroom. She wants to use the same tiles on the floor and all 4 walls and for all the walls to be completely tiled apart from the door. The bathroom is 2.4 metres high, 2 metres wide and 2 metres long, and the door is 2 metres high, 80cm wide and at the end of one of the 4 identical walls. The tiles she wants to use are 40cm x 40cm.
How many of these tiles does she need to tile the whole bathroom?

A) 110 B) 120 C) 135 D) 145 E) 15

Question 4:
Jane and Trevor are both travelling south, from York to London. Jane is driving, whilst Trevor is travelling by train. The speed limit on the roads between York and London is 70mph, whilst the train travels at 90mph. Thus, we should expect that Trevor will arrive first.

Which of the following would weaken this passage's conclusion?

A) The train takes a direct route, whilst the road from York to London goes through several major cities and zig-zags somewhat on its way down the country.
B) Trevor left before Jane.
C) Jane is a conscientious driver, who never exceeds the speed limit.
D) Trevor's train makes a lot of stops on the way, and spends several minutes at each stop waiting for new passengers to board.
E) Meanwhile, Raheem is making the same journey by plane, and will arrive before either Trevor or Jane.

Question 5:
ABC taxis charges a rate of 15p per minute, plus £4. XYZ taxis charges a rate of £4 plus 30p per mile. I live 6 miles from the station.

What would the taxi's average speed have to be on my journey home from the station for the two taxi firms to charge exactly the same fare?

A) 25 B) 30 C) 45 D) 55 E) 60

Question 6:
King Arthur has been issued a challenge by Mordac, his nephew who rules the adjacent Kingdom. Mordac has challenged King Arthur to select a knight to complete a series of challenging obstacles, battling a number of dark creatures along the way, in a test known as the Adzol. The King's squire reports that there are tales told by the elders of the court meaning that only a knight with tremendous courage will succeed in Adzol, and all others will fail. He therefore suggests that Arthur should select Lancelot, the most courageous of all Arthur's Knights. The squire argues that due to what the Elders have said, Lancelot will succeed in the task, but all others will fail.

Which of the following is **NOT** an assumption in the squire's reasoning?

A) Lancelot has sufficient courage to succeed in the Adzol.
B) No other knights in Arthur's command also have tremendous courage, so will all fail Adzol.
C) Great courage is required to be successful in the Adzol.
D) The tales told by the elders of the court are correct.
E) None of the above – they are all assumptions.

Question 7:
Karl is making cupcakes for a wedding. It takes him 25 minutes to prepare each batch of cakes. Only 12 can go in the oven at a time and each batch takes 20 minutes in the oven.

What is the latest time Karl can start if he needs to make 100 cupcakes by 4pm?

A) 11:55am B) 12:20pm C) 12:40pm D) 13:20pm E) 14:00pm

Question 8:

A historian is examining a recently excavated hall beneath a medieval castle. She finds that there are a series of arch-shaped gaps along one length of the wall, surrounded by a different pattern of bricks to that seen elsewhere in the walls. These are found to represent where windows where once located, looking out onto one side of the castle. However, the site is now underground. Underground halls in castles never contain windows, so the historian reasons that this hall must once have been located above the ground. Therefore, the ground level must have changed since this castle was built.

Which of the following represents the main conclusion of this passage?

A) Windows are never found in underground halls.
B) Arch-shaped gaps always indicate that windows were once present.
C) It is unexpected for windows to be found in halls in castles.
D) The hall was once located above ground.
E) The ground level must have changed since this hall was built

Question 9:

The England men's cricket team have recently been knocked out of the world cup after a very poor performance that saw them eliminated at the group stage, managing only 1 win and losing against teams well below them in the rankings. The board of English cricket is sitting down to discuss why the team's performance was so poor, and what can be done to ensure that future world cups have a more positive outcome. The chairman of the board says that the current crop of players is not good enough, and that the team's performance should improve soon, as more able players come through the ranks in the county teams, so no action is needed.

However, the sporting director takes a different view, saying that England have not gone further than the group stage of any cricket world cup for the last 25 years, during which time numerous players have come and gone from the team. The sporting director argues that this long period of poor performance indicates that there is a problem with English cricket, meaning that not enough talented players are being produced in the country. He argues that therefore, steps should be taken to reform English cricket to actively foster the development of more talented players.

Which of the following, if true, would most strengthen the sporting director's argument?

A) The English cricket team is regarded as one of the best in the world, with some of the most talented players.
B) England have been steadily falling lower in the world cricket rankings for the last 25 years, due to poor performances across the board in various cricket competitions.
C) A skilled batsman, who was ranked as the 4th best player in the world, has recently retired from the England team. Now, there are no English cricket players in the top 10 of the world cricket player rankings, which is the first time this has happened in over 70 years.
D) Despite not performing well in world cups, England have performed well in other cricket competitions over the last 20 years.
E) Cricket was invented in England, so everybody expects that England should have a lot of good players in their team

Question 10:
Adam's grandmother has sent him to the shop to buy bread rolls. Usually, bread rolls are 30p for a pack of 6 and so his grandmother has given him the exact amount to buy a certain number of bread rolls. However, today there is a special offer whereby if you buy 3 or more packs of rolls, the price per roll is reduced by 1p. He can now buy 1 more pack than before and get no change.
How many bread rolls was he originally supposed to buying?

A) 4 B) 5 C) 6 D) 24 E) 30

Question 11:

	Boys Absenteeism	Girls Absenteeism	Pupils on Roll	Average
Hazelwood Grammar	7%	Boys' School	300	7%
Heather Park Academy	5%	6%	1000	5.60%
Holland Wood Comprehensive	5%	6%	500	5.60%
Hurlington Academy	Girls' School		200	
Average		7%		

Some of the information is missing from the table above. What is the rate of girls' absenteeism at Hurlington Academy?

A) 6.5% B) 7% C) 9% D) 11.5% E) 13%

Question 12:
Two councillors are considering planning proposals for a new housing estate, to be built on the edge of Bluedown Village. Councillor Johnson argues for a proposal to be built upon brownfield land, land which has previously been built on, rather than greenbelt land, which has not previously been built on. He argues that this will both lower the cost of building the estate, as the land would already have some underlying infrastructure and would not need as much preparation, and will ensure a minimal impact on wildlife around the area.

Which of the following would most weaken the councillor's argument?

A) Brownfield land is often not as appealing as greenbelt land visually, and it is likely that houses built on brownfield land will not sell for as high a price as houses built on greenbelt land.
B) An area of brownfield land on the edge of the village, originally built as an outdoor leisure complex, has since become run down, and ironically is now a haven for various types of rare newts, lizards and birds.
C) Much of the brownfield land around the edge of the village has undergone substantial underground development, with a good system of electricity cables, gas pipes and plumbing in place.
D) The village is surrounded by several greenbelt areas designated as areas of outstanding natural beauty, supporting an abundance of wildlife.
E) The village mayor, who has ultimate control over the planning proposal, agrees with councillor Johnson's argument. Thus, it is likely his recommendations will be followed

Question 13:

Many vegetarians claim that they do not eat meat, poultry or fish because it is unethical to kill a sentient being. Most agree that this argument is logical. However, some Pescatarians have also used this argument, that they do not eat meat because they do not believe in killing sentient beings, but they are happy to eat fish. This argument is clearly illogical. There is powerful evidence that fish fulfil just as much of the criteria for being sentient as do most commonly eaten animals, such as chicken or pigs, but that all these animals lack certain criteria for being "sentient" that humans possess. Thus, pescatarians should either accept the killing of beings less sentient than humans, and thus be happy to eat meat and poultry, or they should not accept the killing of any partially sentient beings, and thus not be happy to eat fish.

Which of the following best illustrates the main **conclusion** of this passage?

A) The argument that it is unethical to eat meat due to not wishing to kill sentient beings but eating fish is acceptable is illogical.
B) Pescatarians cannot use logic.
C) Fish are just as sentient as chicken and pigs, and all these beings are less sentient than humans.
D) It is not unethical to eat meat, poultry or fish.
E) It is unethical to eat all forms of meat, including fish and poultry.

Question 14:

Recent research into cultural attitudes in British has revealed a striking hypocrisy. When asked whether foreign people travelling to British on holiday should learn some English, 60% of respondents answered yes. However, when asked if they would attempt to learn some of the language before travelling to a country which did not speak English, only 15% of the respondents answered yes. This is a shocking double-standard on the part of the British public, and is symptomatic of a deeper underlying issue that British people feel themselves superior to other cultures.

Which of the following can be reliably concluded from this passage?

A) 60% of people in Britain think that foreign people travelling to Britain for a holiday should learn English, but would not learn the language themselves when going on holiday to a country which did not speak English.
B) The British public do not feel that it is important to learn some of the language before travelling to a country which does not speak English.
C) There are numerous issues of racism amongst the British public, stemming from the fact they feel themselves superior to other cultures.
D) Less than 10% of the British public would attempt to learn some of the language before travelling to a country which did not speak English.
E) Some in Britain think that foreign people travelling to Britain for a holiday should learn English, but would not learn the language themselves when going on holiday to a country which did not speak English.

Question 15:

Harriet is a headmistress and she is making 400 information packs for the sixth form open evening. Each information pack needs to have 2 double sided sheets of A4 of general information about the school. She also needs to produce 50 A5 single sided sheets about each of the 30 A Level courses on offer. Single sided A5 costs £0.01 per sheet. Double sided costs twice as much as single sided. A4 printing costs 1.5 times as much as A5.

How much does she spend altogether on the printing?

A) £27 B) £31 C) £35 D) £39 E) £43

Question 16:
Kirkleatham Town football club are currently leading the league. One week they play a crucial match against Redcar Rovers, who are second placed. The points tally of the teams in the table means that if Kirkleatham Town win this game, they will win the league. Before the game, the manager of Kirkleatham Town says that Redcar Rovers are a tough opponent, and that if his team do not play with desire and commitment, they will not win the game. After the game, the manager is asked for comment on the game, and says he was pleased that his team played with so much desire, and showed high levels of commitment. Therefore, Kirkleatham will win the league.

Which of the following best illustrates a flaw in this passage?

A) It has assumed that Kirkleatham will not win the game if they do not play with desire and commitment.
B) It has assumed that if Kirkleatham play with desire and commitment, they will win the game.
C) It has assumed that Kirkleatham played with desire and commitment.
D) It has assumed that Redcar Rovers are a tough opponent, and that Kirkleatham will not be able to easily win the game.
E) It has assumed that if Kirkleatham win the match against Redcar Rovers, they will win the league.

Question 17
Up until the 20th century, all watches were made by hand, by watchmakers. Watchmaking is considered one of the most difficult and delicate of manufacturing skills, requiring immense patience, meticulous attention to detail and an extremely steady hand. However, due to the advent of more accurate technology, most watches are now produced by machines, and only a minority are made by hand, for specialist collectors. Thus, some watchmakers now work for the watch industry, and only perform *repairs* on watches that are initially produced by machines.

Which of the following *cannot* be reliably concluded from this passage?

A) Most watches are now produced by machines, not by hand.
B) Watchmaking is considered one of the most difficult of manufacturing skills
C) Most watchmakers now work for the watch industry, performing repairs on watches rather than producing new ones.
D) The advent of more accurate technology caused the situation today, where most watches are made by machines.
E) Some watches are now made by hand for specialist collectors.

Question 18:
A pizza takeaway is having a sale. If you spend £30 or more at full price, you can get 40% off.
Prices are as follows:

- Basic cheese and tomato pizza: £8 small, £10 large
- All other toppings are £1 each
- Sides are: Garlic bread £3, Potato wedges £2.50, Chips £1.50 and Dips £1 each

Ellie and Mike want to order a large pizza with mushrooms and ham, garlic bread, 2 portions of chips and a dip.

Which of these additional items can they order to minimise the amount they have to pay?

A) Small pizza with pineapple and onion
B) Large pizza with mushroom
C) Barbecue dip
D) 4 portions of potato wedges
E) Garlic bread

Question 19:
The pie chart shows the voting intentions of some constituents interviewed by a polling group, prior to an upcoming election.

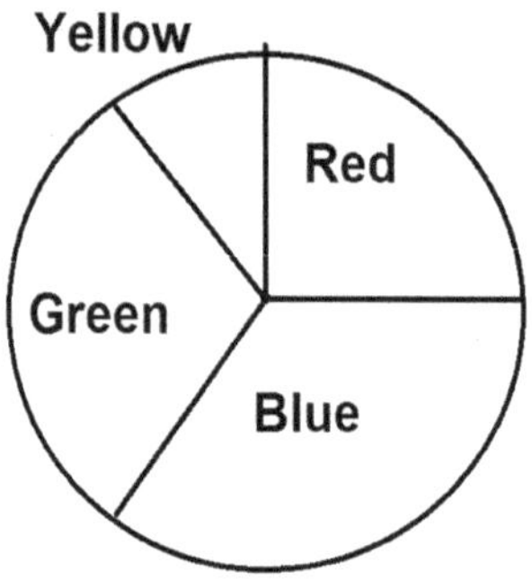

How many times more people said their intention was to vote for the red party than the yellow party?

A) 2 B) 3 C) 4 D) 5 E) 6

Question 20:

	Goals Scored	Goals Conceded
City	10	4
United	8	5
Rovers	1	10

The table above shows the goal scoring record of teams in a football tournament. Each team plays the other teams twice, once at home and once away. Here are the results of the first 4 matches:

- United 2 – 2 City
- Rovers 0 – 3 City
- City 2 – 1 Rovers
- Rovers 0 – 3 United

What were the results of the final two fixtures?

A) United 2 – 0 Rovers, City 0 – 0 United
B) United 1 – 0 Rovers, City 1 – 1 United
C) United 0 – 0 Rovers, City 2 – 1 United
D) United 1 – 0 Rovers, City 2 – 2 United
E) United 2 – 0 Rovers, City 3 – 1 United

Question 21:
Which city-monument pairing is wrong?

A) Barcelona – La Sagrada Familia
B) Amsterdam – Anne Frank house
C) London – the Shard
D) Budapest – Szechenyi Baths
E) Rome – Parthenon

Question 22:
Who painted *'Girl with a Pearl Earring'*?

A) Johannes Vermeer
B) Claude Monet
C) Peter Paul Rubens
D) Vincent van Gogh
E) Rembrandt

END OF SECTION

Section 2

Question 23:
Why do cells undergo mitosis?

1. Asexual Reproduction
2. Sexual Reproduction
3. Growth of the human embryo
4. Replacement of dead cells

A) 1 only
B) 2 only
C) 3 only
D) 4 only
E) 2 and 3
F) 1, 2, and 3
G) 1, 3, and 4
H) 2, 3, and 4

Question 24:
In a healthy person, which one of the following has the highest blood pressure?

A) The vena cava
B) The systemic capillaries
C) The pulmonary artery
D) The pulmonary vein
E) The aorta
F) The coronary artery

The following information applies to questions 25 - 26:

Professor Huang accidentally touches a hot pan and her hand moves away in a reflex action. The diagram below shows a schematic of the reflex arc involved.

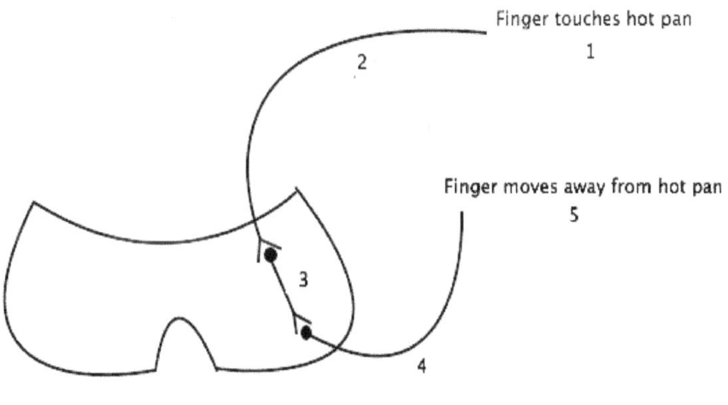

Question 25:
Which option correctly identifies the labels in the pathway?

	Muscle	Sensory Neurone	Receptor	Motor Neurone
A)	1	2	3	4
B)	2	3	1	5
C)	5	2	1	4
D)	1	4	5	2
E)	3	4	5	2
F)	4	2	1	3

Question 26:
Which one of the following statements is correct?

1. Information passes between 1 and 2 chemically.
2. Information passes between 2 and 3 electrically.
3. Information passes between 3 and 4 chemically.

A) 1 only
B) 2 only
C) 3 only
D) 1 and 2
E) 2 and 3
F) 1 and 3
G) All of the above
H) None of the above

Question 27:
For the following reaction, which of the statements below is true?

$6CO_{2\,(g)} + 6H_2O \rightarrow C_6H_{12}O_6 + 6O_{2\,(g)}$

A) Increasing the concentration of the products will increase the reaction rate.
B) Whether this reaction will proceed at room temperature is independent of the entropy.
C) The reaction rate can be monitored by measuring the volume of gas released.
D) This reaction represents aerobic respiration.
E) This reaction represents anaerobic respiration.

The following information applies to questions 28 - 29:

Duchenne muscular dystrophy (DMD) is inherited in an X-linked recessive pattern [transmitted on the X chromosome and requires the absence of normal X chromosomes to result in disease]. A man with DMD has two boys with a woman carrier.

Question 28:
What is the probability that both boys have DMD?

A) 100%
B) 75%
C) 50%
D) 25%
E) 12.5%
F) 0%

Question 29:
If the same couple had two more children, what is the probability that they are both girls with DMD?

A) 100%
B) 75%
C) 50%
D) 25%
E) 12.5%
F) 0%

Question 30:
Which of the following are **NOT** examples of natural selection?

1. Giraffes growing longer necks to eat taller plants.
2. Antibiotic resistance developed by certain strains of bacteria.
3. Pesticide resistance among locusts in farms.
4. Breeding of horses to make them run faster.

A) 1 only
B) 4 only
C) 1 and 3
D) 1 and 4
E) 2 and 4

Question 31:
Which row of the table is correct regarding the cell shown below?

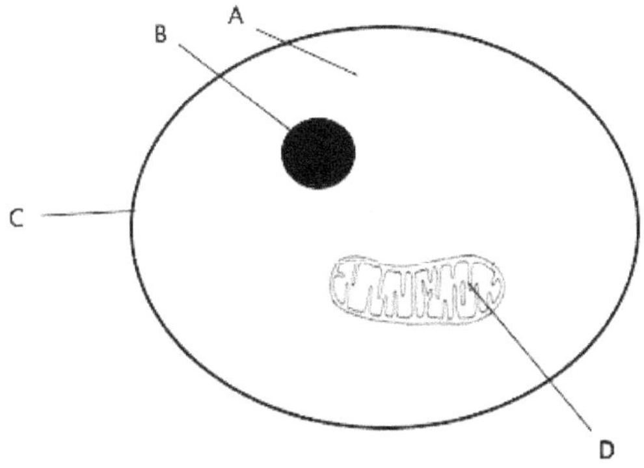

	Most Chemical Reactions occur here	Involved in Energy Release	Cell Type
A)	A	B	Animal
B)	A	B	Bacterial
C)	A	D	Animal
D)	B	D	Bacterial
E)	B	B	Animal
F)	B	A	Bacterial
G)	D	D	Animal
H)	D	B	Bacterial

Question 32:
Which of the following statements about white blood cells is correct?

1. They act by engulfing pathogens such as bacteria.
2. They are able to kill pathogens.
3. They transport carbon dioxide away from dying cells.

A) Only 1
B) Only 2
C) Only 3
D) 1 and 2
E) 2 and 3
F) 1 and 3
G) All
H) None

Question 33:
Which of the following statements are true?

1. Enzymes stabilise the transition state and therefore lower the activation energy.
2. Enzymes distort substrates in order to lower activation energy.
3. Enzymes decrease temperature to slow down reactions and lower the activation energy.
4. Enzymes provide alternative pathways for reactions to occur.

A) 1 only
B) 1 and 2
C) 1 and 4
D) 2 and 4
E) 3 and 4

Question 34:
Which of the following are examples of negative feedback?

1. Salivating whilst waiting for a meal.
2. Throwing a dart.
3. The regulation of blood pH.
4. The regulation of blood pressure.

A) 1 only
B) 1 and 2
C) 3 and 4
D) 2, 3, and 4
E) 1, 2, 3 and 4

Question 35:
Which of the following statements about the immune system are true?

1. White blood cells defend against bacterial and fungal infections.
2. White blood cells can temporarily disable but not kill pathogens.
3. White blood cells use antibodies to fight pathogens.
4. Antibodies are produced by bone marrow stem cells.

A) 1 and 3
B) 1 and 4
C) 2 and 3
D) 2 and 4
E) 1, 2, and 3
F) 1, 3, and 4

Question 36:
The cardiovascular system does **NOT**:

A) Deliver vital nutrients to peripheral cells.
B) Oxygenate blood and transports it to peripheral cells.
C) Act as a mode of transportation for hormones to reach their target organ.
D) Facilitate thermoregulation.
E) Respond to exercise by increasing cardiac output to exercising muscles.

Question 37:
Which of the following statements is correct?

A) Adrenaline can sometimes decrease heart rate.
B) Adrenaline is rarely released during flight or fight responses.
C) Adrenaline causes peripheral vasoconstriction.
D) Adrenaline only affects the cardiovascular system.
E) Adrenaline travels primarily in lymphatic vessels.
F) None of the above.

Question 38:
Which of the following statements is true?

A) Protein synthesis occurs solely in the nucleus.
B) Each amino acid is coded for by three DNA bases.
C) Each protein is coded for by three amino acids.
D) Red blood cells can create new proteins to prolong their lifespan.
E) Protein synthesis isn't necessary for mitosis to take place.
F) None of the above.

Question 39:
A solution of amylase and carbohydrate is present in a beaker, where the pH of the contents is 6.3. Assuming amylase is saturated, which of the following will increase the rate of production of the product?

1. Add sodium bicarbonate
2. Add carbohydrate
3. Add amylase
4. Increase the temperature to 100° C

A) 1 only
B) 2 only
C) 3 only
D) 4 only
E) 1 and 2
F) 1 and 3
G) 1, 2 and 3
H) 1, 3 and 4

Question 40:
Celestial Necrosis is a newly discovered autosomal recessive disorder. A female carrier and a male with the disease produce two boys. What is the probability that neither boy's genotype contains the celestial necrosis allele?

A) 100%
B) 75%
C) 50%
D) 25%
E) 0%

END OF SECTION

Section 3

Question 41:
Which of the following correctly describes the product of the reaction between hydrochloric acid and but-2-ene?

A) CH_3-CH_2-C(Cl)H-CH_3
B) CH_3-C(Cl)-CH_2-CH_3
C) C(Cl)H_2-CH_2-CH_2-CH_3
D) CH_3-CH_2-CH_2-C(Cl)H_2
E) None of the above.

Question 42:
The electrolysis of brine can be represented by the following equation: $2\,NaCl + 2\,X = 2\,Y + Z + Cl_2$
What are the correct formulae for X, Y and Z?

	X	*Y*	*Z*
A)	H_2O	H_2	O_2
B)	H_2O	NaOH	O_2
C)	H_2O	NaOH	H_2
D)	H_2	H_2O	O_2
E)	H_2	NaOH	O_2
F)	H_2	NaOH	H_2
G)	NaOH	H_2O	H_2
H)	NaOH	H_2O	O_2

Question 43:
An unknown element has two isotopes: ^{76}X and ^{78}X. $A_r = 76.5$. Which of the statements below are true of X?

1. ^{76}X is three times as abundant as ^{78}X.
2. ^{78}X is three times as abundant as ^{76}X.
3. ^{76}X is more stable than ^{78}X.

A) 1 only
B) 2 only
C) 3 only
D) 1 and 3
E) 2 and 3
F) None of the above.

Question 44:
For the following reaction, which of the statements below is true?

$6CO_{2\,(g)} + 6H_2O \rightarrow C_6H_{12}O_6 + 6O_{2\,(g)}$

A) Increasing the concentration of the products will increase the reaction rate.
B) Whether this reaction will proceed at room temperature is independent of the entropy.
C) The reaction rate can be monitored by measuring the volume of gas released.
D) This reaction represents aerobic respiration.
E) This reaction represents anaerobic respiration.

Question 45:
Which of the following are true about the formation of polymers?

1. They are formed from saturated molecules.
2. Water is released when polymers form.
3. Polymers only form linear molecules.

A) Only 1
B) Only 2
C) Only 3
D) 1 and 2
E) 1 and 3
F) 2 and 3
G) All of the above.
H) None of the above.

Question 46:
In the reaction between Zinc and Copper (II) sulphate which elements act as oxidising + reducing agents?

A) Zinc is the reducing agent while sulfur is the oxidizing agent.
B) Zinc is the reducing agent while copper in $CuSO_4$ is the oxidizing agent.
C) Copper is the reducing agent while zinc is the oxidizing agent.
D) Oxygen is the reducing agent while copper in $CuSO_4$ is the oxidizing agent.
E) Sulfur is the reducing agent while oxygen is the oxidizing agent.
F) None of the above.

Question 47:
Which of the following statements is true?

A) Acids are compounds that act as proton acceptors in aqueous solution.
B) Acids only exist in a liquid state.
C) Strong acids are partially ionized in a solution.
D) Weak acids generally have a pH or 6 - 7.
E) The reaction between a weak and strong acid produces water and salt.

Question 48:
An unknown element, Z, has 3 isotopes: Z^5, Z^6 and Z^8. Given that the atomic mass of Z is 7, and the relative abundance of Z^5 is 20%, which of the following statements are correct?

1. Z^5 and Z^6 are present in the same abundance.
2. Z^8 is the most abundant of the isotopes.
3. Z^8 is more abundant than Z^5 and Z^6combined

A) 1 only
B) 2 only
C) 3 only
D) 1 and 2 only
E) 2 and 3 only
F) 1 and 3 only
G) 1, 2 and 3
H) None of the statements are correct.

Question 49:
Which of following best describes the products when an acid reacts with a metal that is more reactive than hydrogen?

A) Salt and hydrogen
B) Salt and ammonia
C) Salt and water
D) A weak acid and a weak base
E) A strong acid and a strong base
F) No reaction would occur.

Question 50:
Choose the option which balances the following equation:

a $FeSO_4$ + **b** $K_2Cr_2O_7$ + **c** H_2SO_4 → **d** $(Fe)_2(SO_4)_3$ + **e** $Cr_2(SO_4)_3$ + **f** K_2SO_4 + **g** H_2O

	a	b	c	d	e	f	g
A	6	1	8	3	1	1	7
B	6	1	7	3	1	1	7
C	2	1	6	2	1	1	6
D	12	1	14	4	1	1	14
E	4	1	12	4	1	1	12
F	8	1	8	4	2	1	8

Question 51:
Which of the following statements is correct?

A) Matter consists of atoms that have a net electrical charge.
B) Atoms and ions of the same element have different numbers of protons and electrons but the same number of neutrons.
C) Over 80% of an atom's mass is provided by protons.
D) Atoms of the same element that have different numbers of neutrons react at significantly different rates.
E) Protons in the nucleus of atoms repel each other as they are positively charged.
F) None of the above.

Question 52:
Which of the following statements is correct?

A) The noble gasses are chemically inert and therefore useless to man.
B) All the noble gasses have a full outer electron shell.
C) The majority of noble gasses are brightly coloured.
D) The boiling point of the noble gasses decreases as you progress down the group.
E) Neon is the most abundant noble gas.

END OF SECTION

Section 4

Question 53:
A ball of radius 2 m and density 3 kg/m^3 is released from the top of a frictionless ramp of height 20m and rolls down. What is its speed at the bottom? Take $\pi = 3$ and $g = 10\text{m}^{-2}$.

A) 1 ms^{-1}
B) 4 ms^{-1}
C) 7 ms^{-1}
D) 9 ms^{-1}
E) 14 ms^{-1}
F) 20 ms^{-1}

Question 54:
Which of the following statements is true regarding waves?

A) Waves can transfer mass in the direction of propagation.
B) All waves have the same energy.
C) All light waves have the same energy.
D) Waves can interfere with each other.
E) None of the above.

Question 55:
Rearrange $\frac{(7x+10)}{(9x+5)} = 3z^2 + 2$, to make x the subject.

A) $x = \frac{15\,z^2}{7-9(3z^2+2)}$
B) $x = \frac{15\,z^2}{7+9(3z^2+2)}$
C) $x = -\frac{15\,z^2}{7-9(3z^2+2)}$
D) $x = -\frac{15\,z^2}{7+9(3z^2+2)}$
E) $x = -\frac{15\,z^2}{7+3(3z^2+2)}$
F) $x = \frac{15\,z^2}{7+3(3z^2+2)}$

Question 56:
Element ${}^{188}_{90}X$ decays into two equal daughter nuclei after a single alpha decay and the release of gamma radiation. What is the daughter element?

A) ${}^{91}_{45}D$
B) ${}^{92}_{44}D$
C) ${}^{184}_{88}D$
D) ${}^{186}_{90}D$
E) ${}^{186}_{45}D$

Question 57:
The diagram below shows a series of identical sports fields:

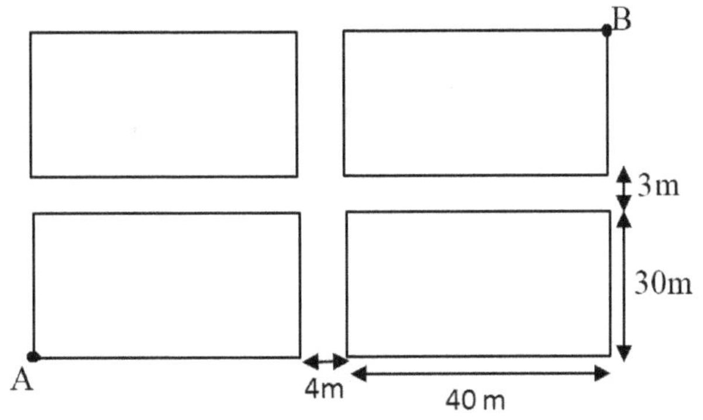

Calculate the shortest distance between points A and B.

A) 100 m
B) 105 m
C) 146 m
D) 148 m
E) 154 m
F) None of the above.

Question 58:

Calculate $\frac{1.25 \times 10^{10} + 1.25 \times 10^{9}}{2.5 \times 10^{8}}$

A) 0
B) 1
C) 55
D) 110
E) 1.25×10^8
F) 5.5×10^7
G) 5.5×10^8

Question 59:

Solve $y = 2x - 1$ and $y = x^2 - 1$ for x and y.

A) (0, -1) and (2, 3)
B) (1, -1) and (2, 2)
C) (1, 4) and (3, 2)
D) (2, -3) and (4, 5)
E) (3, -1) and (3, 1)
F) (4, -2) and (-2, 4)

Question 60:

Tim stands at the waterfront and holds a 30 cm ruler horizontally at eye level one metre in front of him. It lines up so it appears to be exactly the same length as a cruise ship 1 km out to sea. How long is the cruise ship?

A) 299.7 m
B) 300.0 m
C) 333.3 m
D) 29,970 m
E) 30,000 m

END OF PAPER

MOCK PAPER G

Section 1

Question 1:

Irish Folk Band, the Willow, have recently signed a contract with a new manager, and are organising a new musical tour. They and their manager are discussing which country would be best to organise their tour in. The lead singer of the willow would like to organise a tour in Germany, which has a rich history of folk music. However, the new manager finds that ticket sales for folk music concerts in Germany have been steadily declining for several years, whilst France has recently seen a significant increase in ticket sales for folk music concerts. The manager says that this means the group's ticket sales would be higher if they organise a tour in France, than if they organise one in Germany.

Which of the following is an assumption that the manager has made?

A) The band should prioritise profits and organise a tour in the most profitable country possible.
B) The band should not embark upon a new tour and should instead focus on record sales.
C) The decrease of ticket sales in Germany and the increase in France means that the band will sell fewer tickets in Germany than in France.
D) There will not be other countries which are even more profitable than France to organise the tour in.
E) Folk music is popular in France.

Question 2:

A teacher is trying to arrange the 5 students in her class into a seating plan. Her classroom contains 2 tables, arranged one behind the other, which each sit 3 people. Ashley must sit on the front row on the left hand side nearest the board because she has poor eyesight. Bella and Caitlin must not be sat in the same row as each other because they talk and disrupt the class. Danielle needs to be sat next to an empty seat as she sometimes has help from a teaching assistant. Emily should be sat on the end of a row because she has poor mobility and it is hard for her to get into a middle seat.

Who is sitting in the front right seat?

A) Empty B) Bella C) Caitlin D) Danielle E) Emily

Question 3:

Grace and Rose have both been attending an afterschool gymnastics class, which finishes at 5pm. After the class has finished, Grace and Rose cool down and change out of their gym clothes before heading home. Both girls depart at 5:15pm. Grace and Rose both live a 1.5 mile walk away from the local gymnasium. Therefore, they will definitely arrive home at the same time.

Which of the following is **NOT** an assumption made in this argument?

A) Both girls will walk at the same speed.
B) Both girls departed at the same time.
C) The gymnastics class is being held at the local gymnasium.
D) Grace will not get lost on the way home.
E) Both girls are walking home.

Question 4:

Wendy is sending 50 invitations to her housewarming party by first class post. Every envelope contains an invitation weighing 70g, and some who are going to family and friends who live further away also contain a sheet of directions, which weigh 25g. The table below gives the prices of sending letters of certain weights by first or second class post.

If the total cost of sending the invitations is £33, how many of the invitations contain the extra information?

	First Class	Second Class
Less than 50g	£0.50	£0.30
Less than 75g	£0.60	£0.40
Less than 100g	£0.70	£0.50
Less than 125g	£0.80	£0.60
Less than 150g	£0.90	£0.70

A) 15 B) 20 C) 25 D) 30 E) 35

Question 5:

In the Battle of Waterloo, in 1815, French Emperor Napoleon Bonaparte's army was defeated by a British army commanded by British General Arthur Wellesley, Duke of Wellington. Essential to The British army's victory was the arrival of a group of Prussian reinforcements led by Field Marshal Von Blucher, which joined up with The British army and allowed them to overwhelm Bonaparte's left flank. Bonaparte had been aware of the threat posed by Von Blucher's Prussians, and had detached a force of French soldiers several days earlier under the command of Field Marshal Grouchy, with orders to engage the Prussians led by Von Blucher, and prevent them joining up with The British Army.

However, whilst dining at a local inn, Grouchy mistook the sounds of gunfire for thunder, and believed that the battle had been cancelled. He therefore disobeyed his orders and did not engage the Prussians commanded by Von Blucher. Therefore, if Field Marshal Grouchy had not made this mistake and had engaged the Prussian force as commanded, The British would not have won the Battle of waterloo.

Which is the best statement of a flaw in this argument?

A) It implies Field Marshal Grouchy was an incompetent commander, when in fact he was a highly respected general of the day.
B) It assumes that had Grouchy engaged the Prussian force, he would have been able to successfully prevent them joining up with the British army.
C) It assumes that the British army would not have been victorious without the arrival of the Prussian reinforcements.
D) It ignores the other mistakes made by Napoleon which contributed to the British army being victorious in the Battle of Waterloo.
E) It implies that thunder and gunshot sounds are frequently mistaken by generals.

Question 6:

John is a train enthusiast, who has been studying the directions in which trains travel after departing from various London Stations. He finds that Trains departing from King's Cross station in London head North on the East Coast Mainline, and travel to Edinburgh. Trains departing from Waterloo Station head West on the Southwest Mainline and travel to Plymouth. Trains departing from Victoria Station head South and travel to Kent. John surmises that presently, in order to travel on a train from London to Edinburgh, he must get on at King's Cross Station.

Which of the following is an assumption that John has made?

A) The East Coast mainline has the fastest trains.
B) It would not be quicker to take a train from Waterloo to Southampton Airport, then travel to Edinburgh on an Aeroplane.
C) Rail lines will not be built that will allow trains to travel from Waterloo Station or Victoria Station to Edinburgh.
D) King's Cross trains do not have any other destinations other than Edinburgh.
E) There are no other train stations in London from which trains may travel to Edinburgh.

Question 7:

Tanks and armoured vehicles were a hugely influential factor in all battles in World War 2. German tanks were highly superior to the tanks used by France, and this was an essential reason why Germany was able to defeat France in 1940. However, Germany was later defeated in World War 2 by the Soviet Union. Germany lost a number of key battles such as the Battle of Stalingrad and the Battle of Kursk. These victories were essential for the eventual victory of the Soviet Union over Germany. Therefore, the Soviet Union's tanks in the battles of Stalingrad and Kursk must have been superior to those of Germany.

Which of the following is an assumption made in this argument?

A) Tanks were hugely influential in the Battle of Stalingrad.
B) The Battles of Stalingrad and Kursk were essential for the Soviet Union's victory over Germany.
C) The reasons why the Soviet Union defeated Germany in battle were the same as the reasons why Germany defeated France in battle.
D) German tanks being superior to those used by France was an essential reason why Germany was able to defeat France.
E) If the Soviet Union's tanks were superior to Germany's tanks, the Soviet Union's armoured vehicles must also have been superior to Germany's armoured vehicles.

Question 8:

I write my 4 digit pin number down in a coded format, by multiplying the first and second number together, dividing by the third number than subtracting the fourth number. If my code is 3, which of these could my pin number be?

A) 3461 B) 9864 C) 5423 D) 7848 E) 6849

Question 9:

Rental yield for buy to let properties is calculated by dividing the potential rent per year paid for a house by the amount it cost to buy the house and get it in a rentable condition. Tina is considering 5 houses as possible buy to let investments. House A is in good condition and could be rented as it is for £700 a month, and costs £168,000 to buy. House B is also in good condition but is a student house, so Tina would need to buy furniture for it. The house would cost £190,000 to buy and £10,000 to furnish but could be rented for 40 weeks of the year to 4 students at a rent of £125 a week each. House C needs a lot of work doing. It costs £100,000 but would need £44,000 of renovations and would rent for £600 a month. House D costs £200,000 and would need £40,000 of renovations and would rent out for £2000 a month. House E costs £80,000 and would need £20,000 of renovations and could be rented out for £200 a week.

Which house has the highest rental yield?

A) A B) B C) C D) D E) E

Question 10:

Summer and Shaniqua are playing a game of "noughts and crosses". Each player is assigned either "noughts" (O) or "crosses" (X) and they take it in turns to choose an empty box of the 3x3 grid to put their symbol in. The winner is the first person to get a line of 3 of their symbol in any direction in the grid (vertically, horizontally or diagonally). Summer starts the game. The current position is shown below:

X	X	
	O	

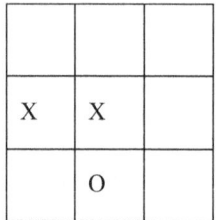

Assuming Shaniqua now plays her symbol in the square which will stop Summer being able to win the game straight away, Summer should play in either of which 2 boxes to ensure she is able to win the game on the next turn no matter what Shaniqua does?

1	2	3
		4
6		5

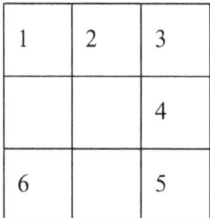

A) 1 and 3 B) 1 and 5 C) 1 and 6 D) 2 and 4 E) 3 and 5

Question 11:

Professors from the department of Pathology at Oxford University are conducting research into possible new treatments for malaria, which is caused by a microbe known as Plasmodium. Research from Sierra Leone, a third world country with a high rate of malaria, has found that liver cells in malaria patients are reactive to the antibody Tarpulin. Plasmodium is known to infect liver cells, and thus liver cells would react to Tarpulin if Plasmodium itself was reactive to Tarpulin. Thus, the professors at Oxford begin to research how Tarpulin can be used to target Plasmodium and treat malaria.

However, this research will not be successful, because liver cells would also react to Tarpulin if the wrong solution is used whilst conducting the experiments. Since malaria is not prevalent in Oxford, the professors must rely on the data from Sierra Leone. If the experiments in Sierra Leone used the wrong solutions, then the liver cells would react to Tarpulin even if Plasmodium does not react to Tarpulin.

Which of the following best illustrates a flaw in this argument?

A) From the fact that Plasmodium infects liver cells, it cannot be inferred that infected liver cells would react to Tarpulin if Plasmodium does.
B) From the fact that the research was carried out in Sierra Leone, it cannot be inferred that the wrong solutions were used.
C) From the fact that the wrong solutions are used, it cannot be inferred that the liver cells would react to Tarpulin.
D) From the fact that Plasmodium is reactive to Tarpulin it cannot be assumed that Tarpulin can be used to combat Plasmodium.
E) From the fact that Liver cells react to Tarpulin, it cannot be inferred that Plasmodium is reactive to Tarpulin.

Question 12:

A cruise ship is sailing from Southampton to Barcelona, making several stops along the way at Calais and Bordeaux, in France, Bilbao in Spain, and Porto in Portugal. At each stop, the ship must wait in a queue to be assigned a Dock at which it can pull in, refuel and resupply. The busier the port, the longer the ship will have to queue to be assigned a Dock. The Captain of the ship is planning the journey, and knows he must work out which ports will have the longest queues.

The Captain made the same journey last year, and found out that Bilbao was the busiest port in Europe during the course of the journey. He also knows that Bordeaux is the busiest port in France, and that Porto is the busiest port in Portugal. Whilst he is planning the journey, he discovers that Calais is busier than Porto. The Captain concludes that he must plan for Bilbao to have the longest queue in the journey, Bordeaux to have the second longest queue, Calais to have the third longest queue, and Porto to have the fourth longest queue.

Which of the following best illustrates a flaw in the Captain's Reasoning?

A) Porto is less busy than Calais, but may be busier than Bordeaux.
B) The rankings may have changed and Bilbao may no longer be the busiest port in Europe.
C) Just because a port is busier does not necessarily mean it will have the longest queues.
D) The ship may not have time to make all the stops.
E) The captain has forgotten to consider how many passengers will embark and disembark at each stop.

Question 13:

A packaging company wishes to make cardboard boxes by taking a flat 1.2 m by 1.2 m square piece of cardboard, cutting square sections out of each corner as shown by the picture below and folding up the sections remaining on each side to make a box. The company experiments with different size boxes by cutting differently sized squares from the corners each time. It makes a box with 10 cm by 10 cm squares cut out of each corner, a box with 20 cm by 20 cm squares cut out of each corner and so on up to one with 50 cm by 50 cm squares cut out of each corner.

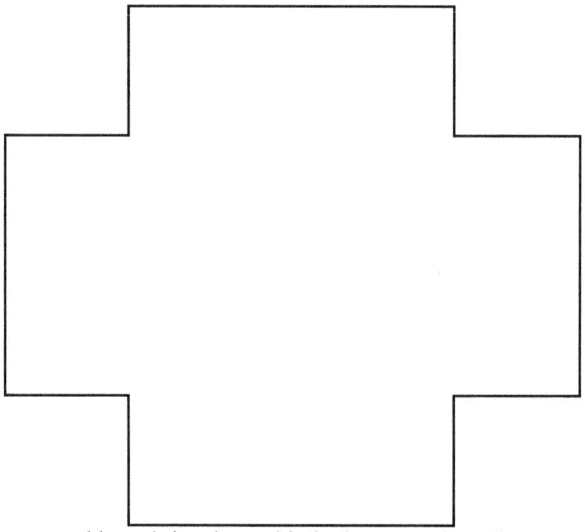

Which side length cut out would result in a box with the largest volume?

A) 10 cm B) 20 cm C) 30 cm D) 40 cm E) 50 cm

Question 14:

The aeroplane was a marvel of modern engineering when it was first developed in the early 20th Century, and was testament to human ingenuity. Throughout the 20th Century, the aeroplane allowed humans to travel more freely and widely than ever before, and allowed people to see and appreciate the stunning natural beauty the world has to offer. However, Aeroplanes also produce lots of pollution, such as Carbon Dioxide and Sulphur Oxide. High levels of Carbon Dioxide in the atmosphere are currently causing global warming, which is destroying or damaging many natural environments throughout the world.

Therefore it is clear that the aeroplane, which once offered such opportunity to appreciate the world's natural beauty, has been largely responsible for damage to various natural environments throughout the world. We must now seek to curb air traffic in order to save the world's remaining natural environments.

Which of the following is the best statement of a flaw in this argument?

A) It assumes that aeroplanes are a major reason for the high levels of Carbon Dioxide in the atmosphere which are currently causing global warming.
B) It assumes that aeroplanes offer greater opportunity to appreciate the world's natural environments.
C) It assumes that high levels of Carbon Dioxide are responsible for global warming.
D) It does not consider the effects of Sulphur Dioxide pollution released by aeroplanes.
E) It implies that we should take action to prevent damage to the world's natural environments.

Question 15:

There has recently been a new election in the UK, and the new government is pondering what policy to adopt on the railway system in the UK. The Chancellor argues that the best policy is to have an entirely privatised railway system, which will encourage different train companies to be competitive, and try and attract customers by providing the best service at the lowest price, thus driving down costs and increasing quality for customers. However, the Transport Minister argues that this is a short-sighted policy. She argues that privatised companies will only run services on the most profitable lines, where there are lots of passengers. Under this system, train companies may not choose to run many services to rural areas. This will lead to rural communities being cut off, with a consequent lack of opportunities for people in these communities. She argues that public funding should be put towards rail services in order to ensure that people in rural communities are adequately served by rail services.

Which of the following, if true, would most strengthen the Transport Minister's argument?

A) The Transport Minister has ultimate power over railway policy, and she can overrule the Chancellor if she sees fit.
B) Many train services to rural communities currently have low passenger numbers, and are unlikely to be profitable.
C) French rail services receive high level of public funding, and users of these services enjoy good quality and low prices.
D) American railway services are privatised with no public funding, and yet rural communities in America are well served by railway services.
E) The Prime Minister agrees with the Transport Minister's line of argument. He sympathises with rural communities and does not believe in a privatised rail system.

Question 16:

Global warming is widely presented in modern society as a cause for significant concern. One particular area often thought to be at risk is the Ice caps of the North and South Poles, which are often presented to be at risk of melting due to increased temperature. Environmentalist groups often campaign for energy consumption to be reduced, thus reducing CO_2 emissions, the leading cause of global warming. However, recent research shows that the North and South Poles are actually becoming cooler, not warmer, thanks to mysterious and unexplained weather patterns. Clearly, high energy consumption is not contributing to damage to the Polar Ice caps.

Which of the following statements can be reliably inferred from this argument?

A) There is no point in reducing energy consumption for environmental reasons.
B) Reducing energy consumption will not reduce CO_2 emissions.
C) We should trust the recent research stating that the North and South poles are becoming cooler.
D) Reducing energy consumption will not contribute to saving the polar ice caps.
E) We should not be concerned about damage to the Polar Ice caps.

Question 17:

Penicillin is one of the major success stories of modern medicine. Since its discovery in 1928, it has grown to become a crucial foundation of medicine, saving countless lives and introducing the age of antibiotics. Alexander Fleming is today given most of the credit for introducing and developing antibiotics, but in fact Fleming played a relatively minor role. Fleming initially discovered Penicillin, but was unable to demonstrate its clinical effectiveness, or discern ways of reliably and consistently producing it. 2 other scientists called Howard Florey and Ernst Chain were actually responsible for developing Penicillin to the point where it could be reliably produced and used in medicine, to treat infections in patients. Clearly, the credit for the wonders worked by Penicillin should not go to Fleming, but to Florey and Chain.

Which of the following best illustrates the main conclusion of this argument?

A) Fleming was unable to develop penicillin to the point of being a viable medical treatment.
B) The credit for Penicillin's effects on medicine should go to Ernst Chain and Howard Florey, not to Alexander Fleming.
C) Without Chain and Florey, Penicillin would not have been developed into a viable treatment.
D) Alexander Fleming only played a small role in the process of Penicillin becoming a feature of modern medicine.
E) Alexander Fleming is not given enough credit for his role in the development of penicillin.

Question 18:

Worcestershire Aquatic Centre is a business seeking to recruit a new dolphin trainer. They interview several candidates, and find that there are 2 candidates which are clearly more suitable than the others. They give both of these candidates a 2nd interview, with further questions about their experience and qualifications.

They discern that Candidate 1 has a proven capability to perform well to crowds, which is likely to bring in more profit to the Aquatic Centre as more people will come and watch a more entertaining dolphin show. However, unlike Candidate 1, Candidate 2 has experience at handling dolphins, and a proven ability to maximise their welfare standards. The manager of the aquatic centre tells the recruiting officer to prioritise profits, and therefore to hire Candidate 1.

Which of the following statements, if true, would most *weaken* the manager's argument?

A) Market research conducted by an external organisation showed that 60% of members of the public would be more likely to attend a dolphin show presented by a charismatic host.
B) Candidate 1's performance experience was not in the aquatic industry.
C) Other aquatic centres with poor welfare standards have been subject to negative media attention and subsequent boycotts.
D) A local charity-run aquatic centre have decided to prioritise donkey welfare and their manager recommends such a strategy.
E) A well-respected business analyst predicts that profit will rise under Candidate 2.

Question 19:

Ancient Egypt was one of the world's most powerful nations for several thousand years, and wondrous structures such as the Sphinxes and the Great Pyramids serve as a permanent reminder of its stature. Many other powerful nations throughout the ages have also built magnificent structures, such as the Colosseum built by the Romans, the Hanging Gardens of Babylon built by the Persians and the Great Wall of China built by the Chinese. As well as building magnificent structures, Rome, Persia and China had one other thing in common, namely a very strong military. Thus, history clearly shows us that in ancient times, for a nation to be a powerful nation, it must have had a very strong military. In addition to building great structures such as the pyramids, Ancient Egypt must have also possessed a very strong military.

Which of the following best illustrates the main conclusion of this argument?

A) In order to be a powerful nation, a nation must build magnificent structures.
B) In Ancient times a very strong military was required to be a powerful nation.
C) Ancient Egypt built magnificent structures; therefore it must have been a powerful nation.
D) Rome, Persia and China were all powerful nations.
E) Ancient Egypt was a powerful nation; therefore it must have had a very strong military.

Question 20:

In 1957 the drug Thalidomide was released, and used to relieve nausea and morning sickness during pregnancy. The pharmaceutical company which released Thalidomide had carried out extensive testing of the drug, and had carried out more tests than was required for new drugs in the 1950s. No adverse affects were reported, and the drug was thought to be safe and effective. However, after it was released, Thalidomide was found to be responsible for severe deformities in thousands of babies whose mothers had taken the drug whilst pregnant with them. When further research was carried out, it was found that the molecules in Thalidomide could adopt 2 molecular structures, known as isomers. One of these isomers was perfectly safe, but the other caused significant biological problems in pregnant women and had been responsible for the deformities in the babies. The company producing Thalidomide had not been aware of this 2nd isomer when developing the drug.

Which of the following is a conclusion that can be drawn from this passage?

A) The company producing Thalidomide had acted irresponsibly by not carrying out the required level of testing for the drug.
B) No isomers of Thalidomide are safe.
C) The drug testing requirements in 1950s were not sufficient to identify all possible isomers of a given drug.
D) Thalidomide was not effective at relieving nausea and morning sickness.
E) The dangerous isomer of Thalidomide was not effective at relieving nausea and morning sickness.

Question 21:

Who wrote '*Republic*'?

A) Aristotle
B) Friedrich Nietzsche
C) Rene Descartes
D) Immanuel Kant
E) Plato

Question 22:

Julian Assange spent 7 years in the London embassy of which country?

A) Russia
B) Ecuador
C) Cuba
D) Australia
E) China

END OF SECTION

Section 2

Question 23:
Which of the following statements are true?

1. Natural selection always favours organisms that are faster or stronger.
2. Genetic variation leads to different adaptations to the environment.
3. Variation is purely due to genetics.

A) Only 1
B) Only 2
C) Only 3
D) 1 and 2
E) 2 and 3
F) 1 and 3
G) All of the above.
H) None of the above.

The following information applies to questions 24 – 25:

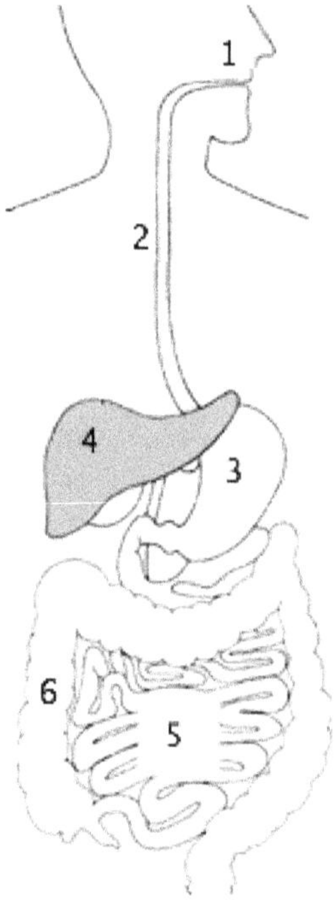

Question 24:
Which of the following numbers indicate where amylase functions?

A) 1 only
B) only
C) 1 and 3
D) 1 and 5
E) 2 and 4
F) 3 and 4
G) 5 and 6

Question 25:
In which of the following does the majority of chemical digestion occur?

A) 1
B) 2
C) 3
D) 4
E) 5
F) 6
G) None of the above.

The following information applies to questions 26-27:
The diagram below shows the genetic inheritance of colour-blindness, which is inherited in a sex-linked recessive manner [transmitted on the X chromosome and requires the absence of normal X chromosomes to result in disease]. X^B is the normal allele and X^b is the colour-blind allele.

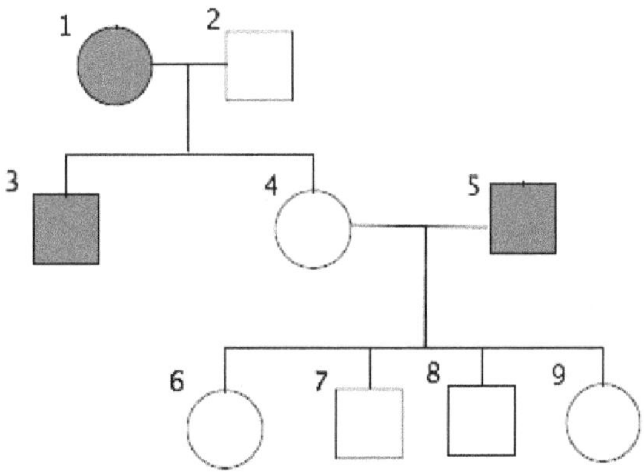

Question 26:
What is the genotype of the individual marked 4?

A) $X^B X^b$ B) $X^B X^B$ C) $X^b X^b$ D) $X^B Y$ E) $X^b Y$

Question 27:
If 8 were to reproduce with a heterozygote female, what is the probability of producing a colour-blind boy?

A) 100%
B) 75%
C) 50%
D) 25%
E) 12.5%
F) 0%

Question 28:
Which of the following correctly describes the passage of urine through the body?

	1st	2nd	3rd	4th
A	Kidney	Ureter	Bladder	Urethra
B	Kidney	Urethra	Bladder	Ureter
C	Urethra	Bladder	Ureter	Kidney
D	Ureter	Kidney	Bladder	Urethra

The following information applies to questions 29 – 30:

In pea plants, colour and stem length are inherited in an autosomal manner. The allele for yellow colour, Y, is dominant to the allele for green colour, y. Furthermore, the allele for tall stem length, T, is dominant to short stem length, t.

When a pea plant of unknown genotype is crossed with a green short-stemmed pea plant, the progeny are 25% yellow + tall-stemmed plants, 25% yellow + short-stemmed plants, 25% green + tall-stemmed plants and 25% green + short-stemmed plants.

Question 29:
What is the genotype of the unknown pea plant?

A) Yytt
B) YyTt
C) YyTT
D) yyTt
E) yyTT
F) yytt

Question 30:
Taking both colour and height into account, how many different combinations of genotypes and phenotypes are possible?

A) 6 genotypes and 3 phenotypes
B) 8 genotypes and 3 phenotypes
C) 8 genotypes and 4 phenotypes
D) 9 genotypes and 4 phenotypes
E) 9 genotypes and 3 phenotypes
F) 10 genotypes and 3 phenotypes

Question 31:
What is the **MOST** important reason for each cell in the human body to have an adequate blood supply?

A) To allow protein synthesis.
B) To receive essential minerals and vitamins for life.
C) To kill invading bacteria.
D) To allow aerobic respiration to take place.
E) To maintain an optimum cellular temperature.
F) To maintain an optimum cellular pH.

Question 32:
Which of the following statements are true?

1. Increasing levels of insulin cause a decrease in blood glucose levels.
2. Increasing levels of glycogen cause an increase in blood glucose levels.
3. Increasing levels of adrenaline decrease the heart rate.

A) 1 only
B) 2 only
C) 3 only
D) 1 and 2
E) 2 and 3
F) 1 and 3
G) 1, 2 and 3

Question 33:
Which of the following rows is correct?

	Oxygenated Blood		Deoxygenated Blood	
A.	Left atrium	Left ventricle	Right atrium	Right ventricle
B.	Left atrium	Right atrium	Left ventricle	Right ventricle
C.	Left atrium	Right ventricle	Right atrium	Right ventricle
D.	Right atrium	Right ventricle	Left atrium	Left ventricle
E.	Left ventricle	Right atrium	Left atrium	Right ventricle

Questions 34-36 are based on the following information:
The pedigree below shows the inheritance of a newly discovered disease that affects connective tissue called Nafram syndrome. Individual 1 is a normal homozygote.

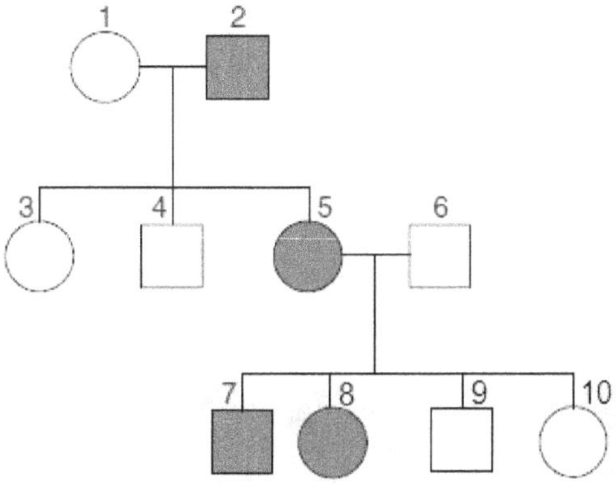

Question 34:
What is the inheritance of Nafram syndrome?

A) Autosomal dominant
B) Autosomal recessive
C) X-linked dominant
D) X-linked recessive
E) Co-dominant

Question 35:
Which individuals must be heterozygous for Nafram syndrome?

A) 1 and 2
B) 8 and 9
C) 2 and 5
D) 5 and 6
E) 6 and 8
F) 6 and 10

Question 36:
Taking N to denote a diseased allele and n to denote a normal allele, which of the following are **NOT** possible genotypes for 6's parents?

1. NN x NN
2. NN x Nn
3. Nn x nn
4. Nn x Nn
5. nn x nn

A) 1 and 2
B) 1 and 3
C) 2 and 3
D) 2 and 5
E) 3 and 4
F) 4 and 5

Question 37:
Which among the following has no endocrine function?

A) The thyroid
B) The ovary
C) The pancreas
D) The adrenal gland
E) The testes
F) None of the above.

Question 38:
Which of the following best describes the passage of blood from the body, through the heart, back to the body?

A) Aorta → Left Ventricle → Left Atrium → Inferior Vena Cava → Right Atrium → Right Ventricle → Lungs
B) Inferior vena cava → Left Atrium → Left Ventricle → Lungs → Right Atrium → Right Ventricle → Aorta
C) Inferior vena cava → Right Ventricle → Right Atrium → Lungs → Left Atrium → Left Ventricle → Aorta
D) Aorta → Left Atrium → Left Ventricle → Lungs → Right Atrium → Right Ventricle → Inferior Vena Cava
E) Right Atrium → Left Atrium → Inferior vena cava → Lungs → Left Atrium → Right Ventricle → Aorta
F) None of the above.

Question 39:
Which of the following best describes the events during inspiration?

	Intrathoracic Pressure	Intercostal Muscles	Diaphragm
A	Increases	Contract	Contracts
B	Increases	Relax	Contracts
C	Increases	Contract	Relaxes
D	Increases	Relax	Relaxes
E	Decreases	Contract	Contracts
F	Decreases	Relax	Contracts
G	Decreases	Contract	Relaxes
H	Decreases	Relax	Relaxes

Question 40:
Which row of the table below describes what happens when external temperature decreases?

	Temperature Change Detected by	Sweat Gland Secretion	Cutaneous Blood Flow
A	Hypothalamus	Increases	Increases
B	Hypothalamus	Increases	Decreases
C	Hypothalamus	Decreases	Increases
D	Hypothalamus	Decreases	Decreases
E	Cerebral Cortex	Increases	Increases
F	Cerebral Cortex	Increases	Decreases
G	Cerebral Cortex	Decreases	Increases
H	Cerebral Cortex	Decreases	Decreases

END OF SECTION

Section 3

Question 41:
Which of the following statements are true about the electrolysis of brine?

1. It describes the reduction of 2 chloride ions to Cl_2.
2. The amount of NaOH produced increases in proportion with the amount of NaCl present in solution, provided there is enough H_2 present to dissolve the NaCl.
3. The redox reaction of the electrolysis of brine results in the production of dissolved NaOH, which is a strong acid.

A) Only 1
B) Only 2
C) Only 3
D) 1 and 2
E) 1 and 3
F) 2 and 3
G) All of the above.
H) None of the above.

Question 42:
Which of the following correctly describes the product of the reaction between propene and hydrofluoric acid (HF)?

A) $C(F)H_3$-CH_2-CH_3
B) CH_3-$C(F)H$-CH_3
C) CH_3-$C(F)H_2$-CH_2
D) CH_3-$C(F)H_2$-CH_3
E) None of the above.

Question 43:
Which of the following are true about the reaction between alkenes and hydrogen halides?

1. The product formed is fully saturated.
2. The hydrogen halide binds at the alkene's saturated double bond.
3. The hydrogen halide forms ionic bonds with the alkene.

A) Only 1
B) Only 2
C) Only 3
D) 1 and 2
E) 2 and 3
F) 1 and 3
G) All of the above.
H) None of the above.

Question 44:
For the following reaction, which of the statements below are true?

$$N_{2(g)} + 3\ H_{2(g)} \rightleftarrows 2\ NH_{3(g)}$$

1. Increasing pressure will cause the equilibrium to shift to the right.
2. Increasing pressure will form more ammonia gas.
3. Increasing the concentration of N_2 will create more ammonia.

A) 1 only
B) 2 only
C) 3 only
D) 1 and 2
E) 2 and 3
F) All of the above.
G) None of the above.

Question 45:
When sodium and chlorine react to form salt, which of the following best represents the bonding and electron configurations of the products and reactants?

	Sodium $_{(s)}$		Chlorine $_{(g)}$		Salt $_{(s)}$	
	Intra-element bond	**Element electron configuration**	**Intra-element bond**	**Element electron configuration**	**Compound bond**	**Compound electron configuration**
A)	Ionic	2, 8, 1	Covalent	2, 8, 8, 1	Ionic	2, 8, 1 : 2, 8, 8, 1
B)	Metallic	2, 7	Covalent	2, 8, 1	Ionic	2, 8 : 2, 8
C)	Covalent	2, 8, 2	Ionic	2, 8, 8	Covalent	2, 8 : 2, 8, 8
D)	Ionic	2, 7	Ionic	2, 8, 8, 7	Covalent	2, 7 : 2, 8, 8, 7
E)	Metallic	2, 8, 1	Covalent	2, 8, 7	Ionic	2, 8 : 2, 8, 8

Question 46:

Which of the following correctly describes the product of the polymerisation of chloroethene molecules?

A

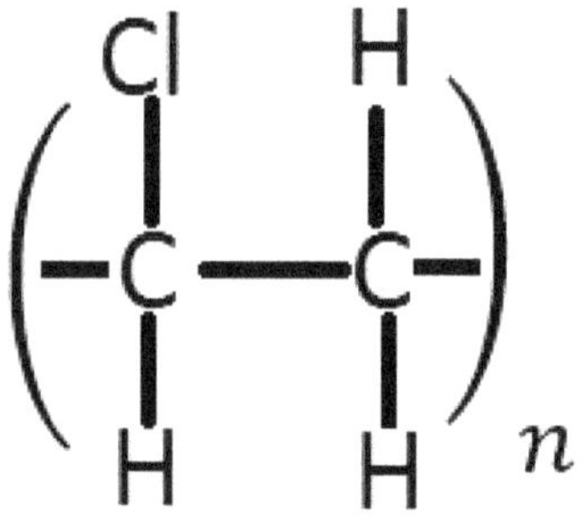

B

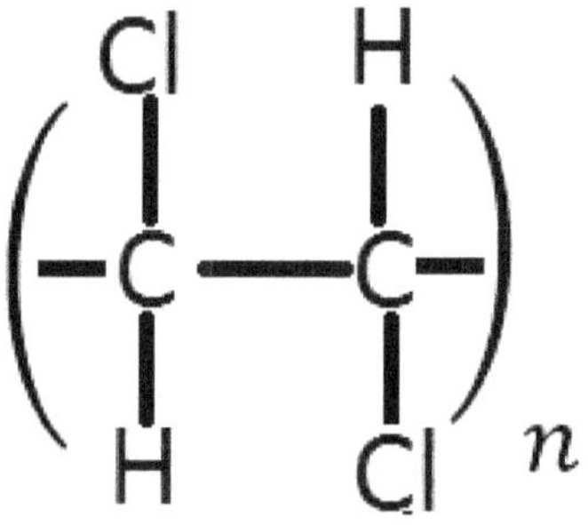

C

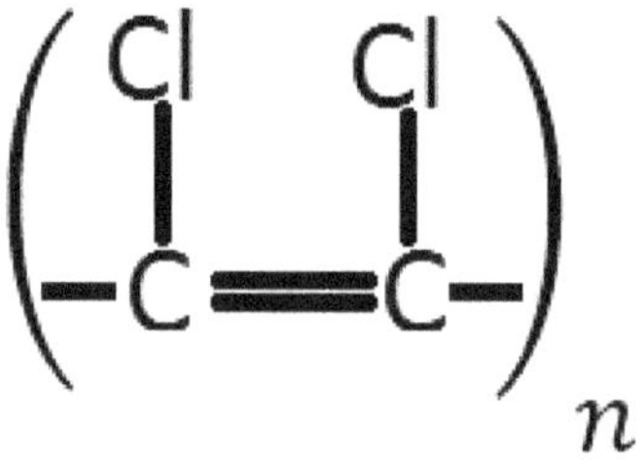

D

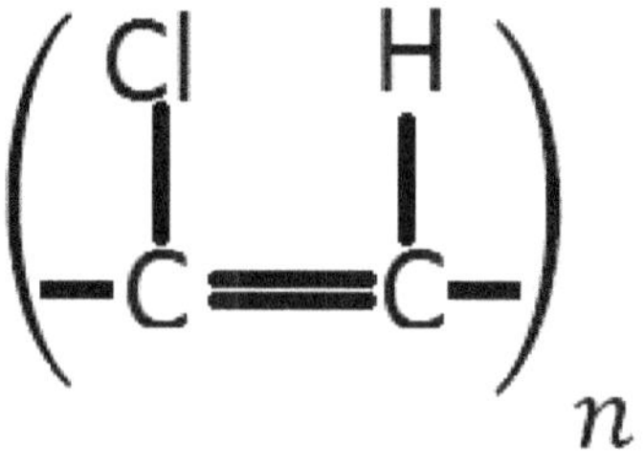

Question 47:
An organic molecule contains 70.6% Carbon, 5.9% Hydrogen and 23.5% Oxygen. It has a molecular mass of 136. What is its chemical formula?

A. C_4H_4O
B. C_5H_4O
C. $C_8H_8O_2$
D. $C_{10}H_8O_2$
E. C_2H_2O

Question 48:
In relation to alkenes, which of the following statements is correct?

1. They all contain double bonds.
2. They can all be reduced to alkanes.
3. Aromatic compounds are also alkenes as they contain double bonds.

A. Only 1
B. Only 2
C. Only 3
D. 1 and 2
E. 2 and 3
F. 1 and 3
G. All of the above.
H. None of the above.

Question 49:
Which of the following statements regarding transition metals is correct?

A. Transition metals form ions that have multiple colours.
B. Transition metals usually form covalent bonds.
C. Transition metals cannot be used as catalysts as they are too reactive.
D. Transition metals are poor conductors of electricity.
E. Transition metals are frequently referred to as f-block elements.

Question 50:
Chlorine is made up of two isotopes, Cl^{35} (atomic mass 34.969) and Cl^{37} (atomic mass 36.966). Given that the atomic mass of chlorine is 35.453, which of the following statements is correct?
A. Cl^{35} is about 3 times more abundant than Cl^{37}.
B. Cl^{35} is about 10 times more abundant than Cl^{37}.
C. Cl^{37} is about 3 times more abundant than Cl^{35}.
D. Cl^{37} is about 10 times more abundant than Cl^{35}.
E. Both isotopes are equally abundant.

Question 51:
20 g of impure Na^{23} reacts completely with excess water to produce 8,000 cm^3 of hydrogen gas under standard conditions. What is the percentage purity of sodium?
[Under standard conditions 1 mole of gas occupies 24 dm^3]

A. 88.0% B. 76.5% C. 66.0% D. 38.0% E. 15.3%

Question 52:
Choose the option which balances the following reaction:

aS + **b**HNO_3 → **c**H_2SO_4 + **d**NO_2 + **e**H_2O

	a	b	c	d	e
A	3	5	3	5	1
B	1	6	1	6	2
C	6	14	6	14	2
D	2	4	2	4	4
E	2	3	2	3	2
F	4	4	4	4	2

END OF SECTION

Section 4

Question 53:
Which of the following statements is **FALSE**?

A) A nuclear power plant may have an accident if free neutrons in a fuel rod aren't captured.
B) Humans cannot currently harness the energy from nuclear fusion.
C) Uncontrolled nuclear fission leads to a large explosion.
D) Mass is conserved during nuclear explosions caused by nuclear bombs.
E) Nuclear fusion produces much more energy than nuclear fission.

Question 54:
Rearrange the following to make m the subject.

$$T = 4\pi\sqrt{\frac{(M+3m)l}{3(M+2m)g}}$$

A) $m = \frac{16\pi^2 lM - 3gMT^2}{48\pi^2 l - 6gT^2}$

B) $m = \frac{16\pi^2 lM - 3gMT^2}{6gT^2 - 48\pi^2 l}$

C) $m = \frac{3gMT^2 - 16\pi^2 lM}{6gT^2 - 48\pi^2 l}$

D) $m = \frac{4\pi^2 lM - 3gMT^2}{6gT^2 - 16\pi^2 l}$

E) $m = \left(\frac{16\pi^2 lM - 3gMT^2}{6gT^2 - 48\pi^2 l}\right)^2$

Question 55:
The mean of a set of 11 numbers is 6. Two numbers are removed and the mean is now 5. Which of the following is not a possible combination of removed numbers?

A. 1 and 20 B. 6 and 9 C. 10 and 11 D. 15 and 6 E. 19 and 2

Question 56:
Which will have a greater current, a circuit with two identical resistors in series or one with the same two resistors in parallel?

A) Series will have greater current than parallel.
B) Parallel will have greater current than series.
C) Same current in both.
D) It depends on the battery.

Question 57:
Evaluate: $\frac{3.4 \times 10^{11} + 3.4 \times 10^{10}}{6.8 \times 10^{12}}$

A) 5.5×10^{-12}
B) 5.5×10^{-2}
C) 5.5×10^{1}
D) 5.5×10^{2}
E) 5.5×10^{10}
F) 5.5×10^{12}

Question 58:
Find the values of angles b and c.

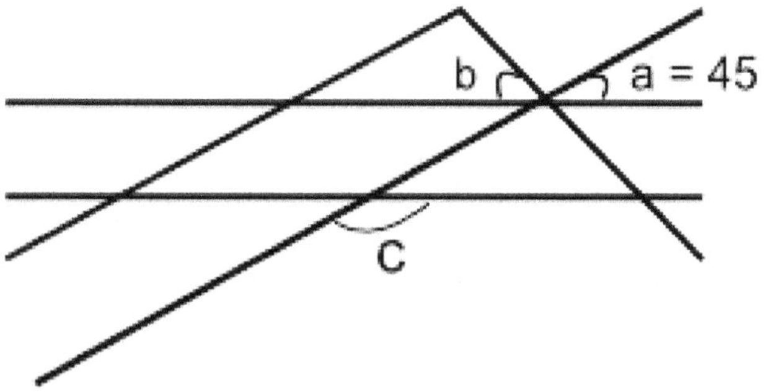

A) 45° and 135°
B) 45° and 130°
C) 50° and 135°
D) 55° and 130°
E) More information needed.

Question 59:
Which of the following statements is true regarding electrolysis?

A) Using an AC-current is most effective.
B) Using a DC-current is most effective.
C) An AC-current causes cations to gather at the cathode.
D) A DC-current would plate the anode in copper from a copper sulphate solution.
E) No current is used in electrolysis.

Question 60:
Evaluate the following expression:
$((\frac{6}{8} \text{x} \frac{7}{3}) \div (\frac{7}{5} \text{x} \frac{2}{6}))$ x 0.40 x 15% x 5% x π x $(\sqrt{e^2})$ x 0.20 x $(e\pi)^{-1}$

A) $\frac{4}{55}$
B) $\frac{8}{770}$
C) $\frac{9}{4{,}000}$
D) $\frac{8}{54{,}321}$
E) $\frac{9}{67{,}800}$

END OF PAPER

MOCK PAPER H

Section 1

Question 1:

A chemical change may add something to a substance, or subtract something from it, or it may both subtract and add, making a new substance with entirely different properties. Sulphur and carbon are two stable solids. The chemical union of the two forms a volatile liquid. A substance may be at one time a solid, at another a liquid, at another a gas, and yet not undergo any chemical change, because in each case the chemical composition is identical.

Which of the following statements cannot be reliably concluded from the above passage?

A) The chemical composition of a compound may influence its physical nature.
B) Substances can exist as solid, liquid or gas, without their chemical composition changing.
C) Chemicals can be combined to create a new substance with similar or very different properties.
D) Combining two substances in one state can lead to the production of a compound in a completely different state.
E) The transition from solid to liquid is not a chemical one.

Question 2:

In the sequence B Y F U I R K P ? ? Which two letters come next?

A) U N B) M N C) L O D) H O E) N M

Question 3:

An insect differs from a horse, for example, as much as a modern printing press differs from the press Franklin used. Both machines are made of iron, steel, wood, etc., and both print; but the plan of their structure differs throughout, and some parts are wanting in the simpler press, which are present and absolutely essential in the other. So with the two sorts of animals; they are built up originally out of protoplasm, or the original jelly-like germinal matter, which fills the cells composing their tissues, and nearly the same chemical elements occur in both, but the mode in which these are combined, the arrangement of their products: the muscular, nervous and skin tissues, differ in the two animals.

Which of the following statements can be reliably concluded from the above passage?

A) The printing press has adapted from the press Franklin used, due to the designers observing differences in nature.
B) Horses and insects differ as they are made up of completely different chemical elements.
C) The muscular, nervous and skin tissues are what define an organism.
D) Chemical elements make up protoplasm, which is the building block for all major organisms.
E) It is the manner in which chemicals are arranged that determine an organism as a final product.

Question 4:

What day comes two days after the day, which comes four days after the day, which comes immediately after the day, which comes two days before Monday?

A) Monday B) Tuesday C) Thursday D) Saturday E) Sunday

Question 5:
Cellulose is distinguished by its inherent constructive functions, and these functions take effect in the plastic or colloidal condition of the substance. These properties are equally conspicuous in the synthetical derivatives of the compound.

Which of the following statements would weaken the above passage?

A) Cellulose has a constructive role in nature.
B) Synthetic cellulose is made from natural cellulose.
C) Synthetic and natural cellulose are structurally very similar.
D) Synthetic cellulose only actually shares some of its properties with natural cellulose.
E) Synthetics cellulose is more useful in industry than natural cellulose.

Question 6:
If John gives Michael £20, the ratio of their money is 2:1. If Michael gives John £5, the ratio of John's money to Michael's is 5:1. How much money do they have combined?

A) £180 B) £120 C) £90 D) £210 E) £150

Question 7:
From the primitive pine-torch to the paraffin candle, how wide an interval! Between them how vast a contrast! The means adopted by man to illuminate his home at night, stamp at once his position in the scale of civilisation. The fluid bitumen of the far East, blazing in rude vessels of baked earth; the Etruscan lamp, exquisite in form, yet ill adapted to its office; the whale, seal, or bear fat, filling the hut of the Esquimaux or Lap with odour rather than light; the huge wax candle on the glittering altar, the range of gas lamps in our streets, all have their stories to tell.

Which of the following statements best summarises the above passage?

A) Burning animal fat was the original way to produce fire.
B) The use of fire has spread to all corners of the Earth.
C) Using fire for light is what defines us as being human.
D) Each light source over the globe is able to tell its own tale.
E) The development and evolution of the use of fire helps to define mankind as a civilisation.

Question 8:
972 patients ordered food for lunch. They could choose roast chicken, mac and cheese, vegetable chilli or cottage pie. Half chose the roast chicken, 1/3 chose the mac and cheese and 1/12 chose the cottage pie.

How many opted for the vegetarian option?
A) 81 B) 92 C) 68 D) 95 E) 102

Question 9:
It was a little late to search for the philosophers' stone in 1669, yet it was in such a search that phosphorus was discovered. Wilhelm Homberg (1652-1715) described it in the following manner: "a man little known, of low birth, with a bizarre and mysterious nature in all he did, found this luminous matter while searching for something else."

What can be reliably concluded about the above passage?

A) Phosphorous was easy to identify as a result of its luminous nature.
B) Phosphorous was found as a result of this man's low social status.
C) Phosphorous was identified by accident, in the search for the philosophers' stone.
D) Wilhelm Homberg discovered phosphorous.
E) Phosphorous was discovered in the 18th century.

Question 10:
How many minutes past noon is it, if 3 times this many minutes before 3pm is 28 minutes later than this many minutes past noon?

A) 54 B) 32 C) 45 D) 38 E) 18

Question 11:
Everyone is familiar with the main facts of such a life-story as that of a moth or butterfly. The form of the adult insect is dominated by the wings—two pairs of scaly wings, carried respectively on the middle and hindmost of the three segments that make up the *thorax* or central region of the insect's body. Each of these three segments carries a pair of legs.

Which of the following statements can be concluded from the above statement?

A) The wings of the insects alternate patterns when the insect flies.
B) The wings that attach to the segments of the insect's body are the most prominent feature of the butterfly or moth.
C) Wings attach to each of the three segments of the thorax.
D) Moths and butterflies are very similar in that each segment of their thorax carries a pair of legs.
E) Scaly wings protect these creatures from predators.

Question 12:
In 2007 AD, Halley's Comet and Comet Encke were observed in the same calendar year. Halley's Comet is observed on average once every 73 years; Comet Encke is observed on average once every 104 years. Based on this, estimate the calendar year in which both Halley's Comet and Comet Encke are next observed in the same year.

A) 9559 AD B) 2114 AD C) 5643 AD D) 3562 AD E) 1757 AD

Question 13:
In a school there are 40 more girls than there are boys. The boys make up a percentage of 40% of the school. What is the number of students in the school?

A) 150 B) 200 C) 300 D) 500 E) 720

Question 14:
5 cars are travelling down a road in a line. The red car is following the blue car; the yellow car is in front of the green car. The purple car is between the green car and the blue car. What colour is the car second in line?

A) Red B) Blue C) Yellow D) Green E) Purple

Question 15:
To get to school, Joanne takes the school bus every morning. If she misses this, then she can take the public bus to school. The school bus arrives at 08:15, which if she misses will come again at 08:37. The public bus comes every 17 minutes, starting at 06:56. The school bus takes 24 minutes to get to her school; the public bus takes 18 minutes. If she arrives at the bus stop at 08:25, which bus must she catch to get to school first?

A) The 08:37 school bus
B) The 08:26 public bus
C) The 08: 38 public bus
D) The 08: 31 public bus

Question 16:
Puddle ducks are typically birds of fresh, shallow marshes and rivers rather than of large lakes and bays. They are good divers, but usually feed by dabbling or tipping rather than submerging. The speculum, or coloured wing patch, is generally iridescent and bright, and often a tell-tale field mark. Any duck feeding in croplands will likely be a puddle duck, for most of this group are sure-footed and can walk and run well on land. Their diet is mostly vegetable, and grain-fed mallards or pintails or acorn-fattened wood ducks are highly regarded as food.

Which of the following statements summarises the above passage best?

A) Other ducks are often eaten by puddle ducks in both large lakes and shallower waters.
B) Puddle ducks feed mainly without diving to gain vegetarian food sources.
C) Puddle ducks are the most common duck seen in croplands because they are vegetarian.
D) Other ducks are prone to predate on puddle ducks.
E) Puddle ducks live in large lakes as they can access vegetable food sources easily.

Question 17:

When the earth had to be prepared for the habitation of man, a veil, as it were, of intermediate being was spread between him and its darkness, in which were joined, in a subdued measure, the stability and the insensibility of the Earth, and the passion and perishing of mankind.

Which of the following statements best summarises the above statement?

A) The veil discussed is what links the good and evil of the human race.
B) Without this veil, mankind would not exist.
C) The Earth has more good than evil.
D) The veil keeps the human race alive.
E) Mankind would be better off without such a veil.

Question 18:
What is the value of ? in the following sequence:
3 1 6 8
8 4 5 0
4 2 7 8
9 2 3 ?

A) 5 B) 4 C) 8 D) 2 E) 7

Question 19:

Metformin has been thought to inhibit the process of fat cell growth. This is because *in vitro* metformin causes fat cells to stop growing. However, when a metformin inhibitor is used alongside metformin, the fat cells still don't grow. Thus we can conclude that metformin does not inhibit fat cell growth.

Which of the following statements highlights the flaw in the argument?

A) Metformin doesn't inhibit fat cell growth.
B) The mechanism by which metformin inhibits fat cell growth is poorly understood.
C) We are not aware of how this inhibitor acts to inhibit the actions of metformin.
D) Fat cell growth has not been quantified here.
E) Metformin does not inhibit fat cell growth *in vivo.*

Question 20:

All dancers are strong. Some dancers are pretty. Alexandra is strong, and Katie is pretty.

Choose a correct statement

A) Alexandra is a dancer
B) Katie is not a dancer
C) A dancer can be strong and pretty
D) A dancer can be strong and ugly

Question 21:

Who wrote *Micrographia*?

A) Antonie van Leeuwenhoek
B) Robert Boyle
C) Galileo
D) Robert Hooke
E) Isaac Newton

Question 22:

When did the Arab Spring occur?

A) 2010-12
B) 2016-18
C) 2004-6
D) 2008-10
E) 1997-99

END OF SECTION

Section 2

Question 23:

Hydrogen Bicarbonate (HCO_3^-) acts as a buffer in the blood i.e. to keep the PH close to 7.

Which statement is true regarding bicarbonate?

A) It is alkaline.
B) It is an acidic molecule.
C) If the pH of the blood drops below 7, bicarbonate will release the H^+ ion to stabilise the pH.
D) It is only released when the pH drops below 7.
E) It is bound to protein in the blood.

Question 24:

The below statements are about breathing. Which of them are correct?

1. The diaphragm plays no part in breathing.
2. The intercostal muscles relax during exhalation to allow the ribcage to move inwards and downwards.
3. The total pressure inside the chest decreases relative to the pressure outside the body during inhaling to draw air inside the lungs.

A) 1 only
B) 2 only
C) 3 only
D) 2 and 3
E) 1 and 3
F) None

Question 25:

In pregnancy the foetus is supplied with blood from the mother via the umbilical cord. This cord is comprised of one vein and two arteries. The table below shows which vessel carries which type of blood in which direction.

Vessel	Direction	Blood
1. Vein	Mother to foetus	Oxygenated
2. Artery	Foetus to Mother	Deoxygenated
3. Artery	Foetus to Mother	Oxygenated
4. Vein	Mother to Foetus	Deoxygenated

Which options are correct?

A) 1 only
B) 2 only
C) 3 only
D) 4 only
E) 1 and 2
F) 2 and 3
G) 4 and 1
H) 3 and 1

Question 26:

What is the function of the kidneys?

1. Ultrafiltration
2. Kill bacteria in the blood
3. Reabsorption
4. Release of waste
5. Store water
6. Produce hormones
7. Blood glucose regulation

A) 1 only
B) 2 only
C) 3 only
D) 4 only
E) 5 only
F) 6 and 7
G) 3 and 5
H) 1, 3 and 4
I) 4, 5 and 6

Question 27:
Mike and Vanessa are two healthy adults. They have two children. Their first child, Rory, was born with Haemophilia B, an X linked recessive disorder that causes problems with blood clotting. They have just had another baby, a girl and want to get her tested for the condition. What is the likelihood of the baby girl having the condition?

A) 0% B) 25% C) 50% D) 75% E) 34%

Question 28:
Bacteria invade the body and produce toxins that kill cells.

What are some of the first line defences the body has to prevent bacteria entering?
1. Mucus lining the airways
2. Heat produced by the body
3. Skin
4. Antibodies produced by the immune system
5. Toxins produced by the body
6. Hydrochloric acid in the stomach

A) 1 only
B) 2 only
C) 3 only
D) 1, 3, 4 and 6
E) 4, 5 and 6
F) 1, 3 and 6
G) 2 and 4

Question 29:
Which of the following is true with regards to osmosis?

A) It does not require a concentration gradient
B) It can apply to any substance, not just water
C) It is the movement of water across a partially permeable membrane
D) It is an active process
E) Transporters move water molecules across the membrane of cells

Question 30:
The carbon cycle is the cycle regarding the intake and release of carbon by organisms. Which of these statements are true?

A) Plants take carbon via photosynthesis and taking nutrients from the soil, which have come from decayed organisms.
B) Animals give off carbon via respiration, waste, eating and death.
C) The CO_2 in the air comes from burning of plant/animal products and respiration from living organisms only.
D) Trees do not store any carbon as they give it all off as carbon dioxide.

Question 31:
Enzymes are thought to work by two mechanisms – lock and key or the induced fit theory. The Lock and Key theory states that the active site of an enzyme is already perfectly shaped for the substrate, whereas the induced fit theory states that the enzyme's active site moulds itself around the substrate's shape. Which of these statements is true?

A) Enzymes are substrate specific.
B) The induced fit theory allows multiple, different types of substrates to be acted on by one enzyme.
C) The induced fit theory allows multiple, different types of enzymes to work on the same substrate.
D) The lock and key theory does not allow space for catatonic reactions (breaking the substrate up.

Questions 32-33 are based on the following information:
DNA is made up of the four nucleotide bases: adenine, cytosine, guanine and thymine. A triplet repeat or codon is a sequence of three nucleotides which code for an amino acid. While there are only 20 amino acids there are 64 different combinations of the four DNA nucleotide bases. This means that more than one combination of 3 DNA nucleotides sequences code for the same amino acid.

Question 32:
Which property of the DNA code is described above?

A) The code is unambiguous.
B) The code is universal.
C) The code is non-overlapping.
D) The code is degenerate.
E) The code is preserved.
F) The code has no punctuation.

Question 33:
Which type of mutation does the described property protect against the most?
A) An insertion - where a single nucleotide is inserted.
B) A point mutation - where a single nucleotide is replaced for another.
C) A deletion - where a single nucleotide is deleted.
D) A repeat expansion - where a repeated trinucleotide sequence is added.
E) A duplication - where a piece of DNA is abnormally copied.

Question 34:

Which of the following processes involve active transport?

1. Reabsorption of glucose in the kidney.
2. Movement of carbon dioxide into the alveoli in the lungs.
3. Movement of chemicals in a neural synapse.

A) 1 only
B) 2 only
C) 3 only
D) 1 and 2
E) 1 and 3
F) 2 and 3
G) 1, 2 and 3

Question 35:
Which of the following statements is correct about enzymes?

A) All enzymes are made up of amino acids only.
B) Enzymes can sometimes slow the rate of reactions.
C) Enzymes have no impact on reaction temperatures.
D) Enzymes are heat sensitive but resistant to changes in pH.
E) Enzymes are unspecific in their substrate use.
F) None of the above.

Question 36:
Which of the following statements about the Krebs cycle are correct?

1. Three molecules of reduced NAD and one molecule of reduced FAD are produced each turn
2. Citric acid is regenerated to be used in the next cycle
3. ATP can be produced by substrate-level phosphorylation

A) 1
B) 2
C) 3
D) 1 and 2
E) 1 and 3
F) 1, 2 and 3

Question 37:
Which of the following statements about the light-dependent reaction are correct?

1. Cyclic phosphorylation uses photosystems I and II
2. Non-cyclic phosphorylation produces ATP, NADPH and oxygen
3. Water is required for both cyclic and non-cyclic photophosphorylation

A) 1
B) 2
C) 3
D) 1 and 2
E) 1 and 3
F) 1, 2 and 3

Question 38:
Which of the following statements about the Calvin cycle are correct?

1. RUBISCO is a co-enzyme
2. It requires 6 turns of he Calvin cycle to make 1 glucose molecules
3. Fatty acids can be synthesised from glycerate-3-phosphate

A) 1
B) 2
C) 2 and 3
D) 1 and 3
E) 1, 2 and 3
F) None of them

Question 39:
Which of the following statements about action potentials are correct?

1. Depolarisation is driven by an influx of sodium ions
2. Hyperpolarisation makes action potentials unidirectional
3. The speed of an action potential depends on the temperature and the diameter of the axon

A) 1
B) 2
C) 3
D) 1 and 2
E) 1 and 3
F) 1, 2 and 3

Question 40:
A patient has been diagnosed with type 1 diabetes. Which statements about hormonal control of glucose are correct?

1. Insulin injections need to be closely monitored to prevent hypoglycaemia
2. Adrenaline increases the storage of glucose as glycogen
3. Glucagon is released from α-cells of the pancreas in response to a fall in blood glucose

END OF SECTION

Section 3

Question 41:

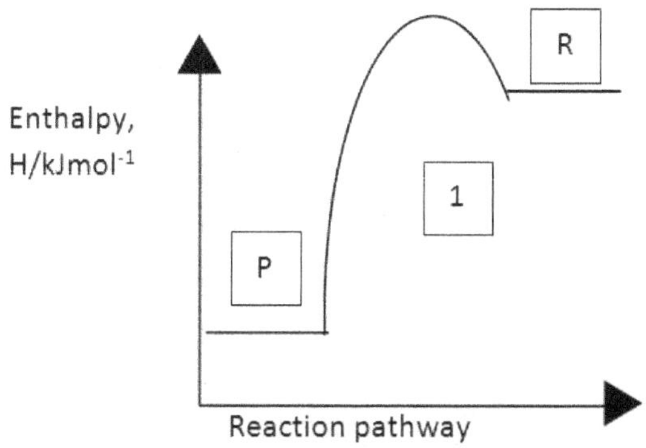

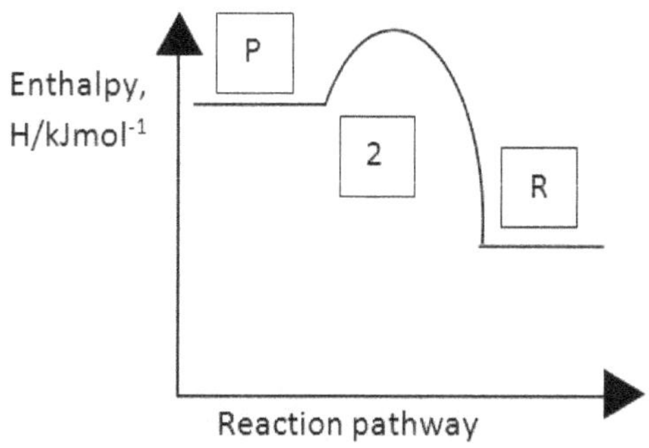

The two graphs shown above are Enthalpy profile diagrams. Which best describes an endothermic reaction?

	Graph	ΔH	Heat energy	Stability of reactants
A)	1	Negative	Absorbed from surroundings	P is more stable than R
B)	2	Negative	Released to surroundings	R is more stable than P
C)	1	Positive	Absorbed from surroundings	P is more stable than R
D)	2	Positive	Absorbed from surroundings	R is more stable than P

Question 42:
Pyrite, also known as Fool's Gold, is an ore of Iron containing sulphur in the form of iron (II) disulphide, FeS_2. By mass 75% of this ore is FeS_2.

Calculate the maximum mass of iron that can be extracted from 480kg of ore.
[A_r: Fe = 55; S = 32]

A) 167.7kg B) 200kg C) 360.5kg D) 118kg E) 120.2kg

Question 43:
$X_{(s)} + FeSO_{4(aq)} \rightarrow XSO_{4(aq)} + Fe_{(S)}$

Which metal can be correctly be substituted in X's place?

A) Tin (Sn)
B) Zinc (Zn)
C) Lead (Pb)
D) Silver (Ag)
E) Copper (Cu)

Question 44:
Which of the following statements about catalysts are true?

1. Catalysts reduce the energy required for a reaction to take place.
2. Catalysts are used up in reactions.
3. Catalysed reactions are almost always exothermic.

A. 1 only B. 2 only C. 1 and 2 D. 2 and 3 E. 1, 2 and 3

Question 45:

The element shown below is Germanium. It has an ionic charge of 4+. How many electrons does one atom of Germanium have?

73
Ge
32

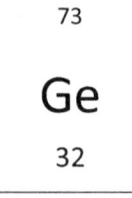

A) 32 B) 73 C) 36 D) 41 E) 4

Question 46:

For the following reaction, which of the statements is true?

$CH_{4(g)} + 2O_{2(g)} \rightarrow 2H_2O_{(aq)} + CO_{2(g)}$

A) This is an example of complete combustion.
B) By increasing the concentration of CO_2 you can increase the rate of combustion
C) The reaction is anaerobic
D) Combustion of a gas always produces a liquid like water
E) If you remove some of the oxygen you get more product.

Question 47:

Which of the following statements is true?

2. Ethane and ethene can both dissolve in organic solvents.
3. Ethane and ethene can both be hydrogenated in the presence of Nickel.
4. Breaking C=C requires double the energy needed to break C-C.

A. 1 only
B. 2 only
C. 3 only
D. 1 and 2 only
E. 2 and 3 only
F. 1 and 3 only
G. 1, 2 and 3

Question 48:

Diamond, Graphite, Methane and Ammonia all exhibit covalent bonding. Which row adequately describes the properties associated with each?

	Compound	Melting Point	Able to conduct electricity	Soluble in water
1.	Diamond	High	Yes	No
2.	Graphite	High	Yes	No
3.	$CH_{4\,(g)}$	Low	No	No
4.	$NH_{3\,(g)}$	Low	No	Yes

A. 1 and 2 only
B. 2 and 3 only
C. 1 and 3 only
D. 1 and 4 only
E. 1, 2 and 3
F. 2, 3 and 4
G. 1,2 and 4
H. 1, 2, 3 and 4

Question 49:

What is the name of the molecule below?

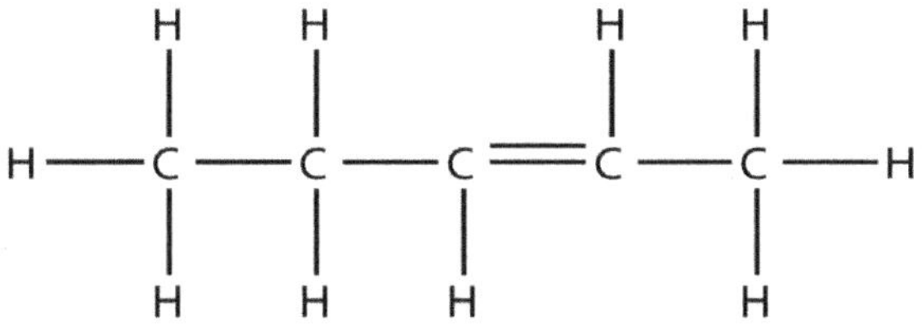

A. But-1-ene
B. But-2-ene
C. Pent-3-ene
D. Pent-1-ene
E. Pent-2-ene
F. Pentane
G. Pentanoic acid

Question 50:

Which of the following statements is correct regarding Group 1 elements? [Excluding Hydrogen]

A. The oxidation number of Group 1 elements usually decreases in most reactions.
B. Reactivity decreases as you progress down Group 1.
C. Group 1 elements do not react with water.
D. All Group 1 elements react spontaneously with oxygen.
E. All of the above.
F. None of the above.

Question 51:

Which of the following statements about electrolysis are correct?

1. The cathode attracts negatively charged ions.
2. Atoms are reduced at the anode.
3. Electrolysis can be used to separate mixtures.

A. Only 1
B. Only 2
C. Only 3
D. 1 and 2
E. 2 and 3
F. 1 and 3
G. 1, 2 and 3
H. None of the above.

Question 52:

Which of the following is **NOT** an isomer of pentane?

A. $CH_3CH_2CH_2CH_2CH_3$
B. $CH_3C(CH_3)CH_3CH_3$
C. $CH_3(CH_2)_3CH_3$
D. $CH_3C(CH_3)_2CH_3$

END OF PAPER

Section 4

Question 53:

Which of the statements regarding this series circuit is true?

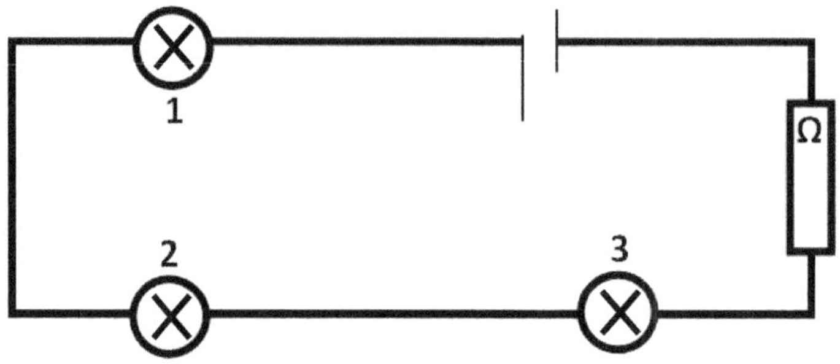

A) Current is different at different points in the circuit.
B) Potential difference is shared between the three lightbulbs.
C) Resistance is constant throughout the circuit.
D) The current is higher in bulb 1 than in bulbs 2 and 3.

Question 54:
Bill wants to lay down laminate flooring in his living room, which has an in-built circular fish tank that he will have to lay the flooring around. He has decided to buy planks that he can cut to fit the dimensions of his room. He must, however, buy whole planks and cut them down himself. The room's dimensions are given below, as are those of one plank.

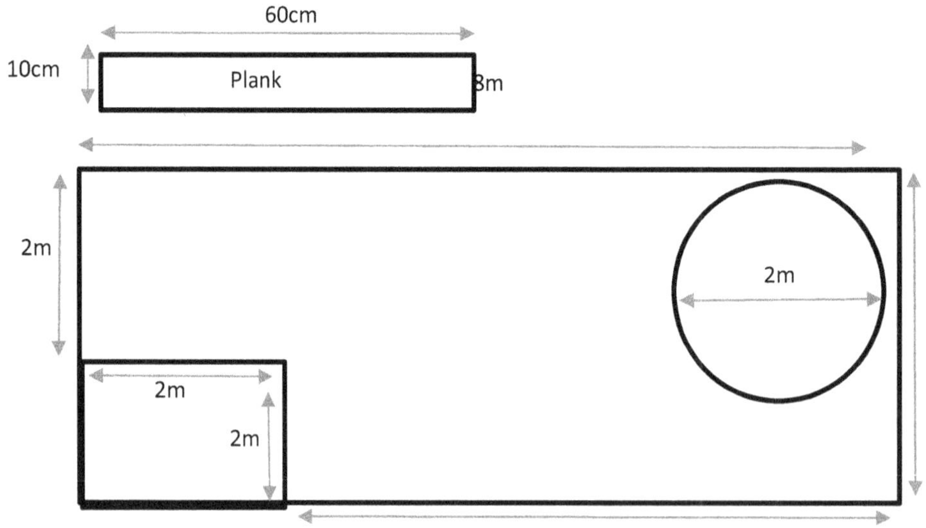

Calculate the number of planks needed to cover the whole floor. Take $\pi = 3$.

A) 30 B) 417 C) 600 D) 589 E) 43

Question 55:
Solve $y = x^2 - 3x + 4$ and $y - x = 1$ as (x,y).

A) (-1, 2) and (3,4)
B) (1,2) and (3,4)
C) (7,-2) and (6,5)
D) (2,-3) and (4,-1)
E) (1,-1) and (-7,-1)

Question 56:
A ball of mass 5kg is at rest at the top of a 5m slope. Calculate the velocity of the ball as it travels down the slope. Take $g = 10kgm^{-1}$ and assume there is no resistance.

A) 10 B) 45 C) 100 D) 5 E) 6

Question 57:
Which of the following statements is true regarding Red Shift?

A) The further a distant galaxy or celestial object is, the further down the red end of the light spectrum it's light will be.
B) The closer a galaxy gets, the longer it's wavelengths get, thus moving down the red end of the spectrum.
C) Red shift means that we never see the real light from distant galaxies.
D) We can never tell how far away galaxies are using red shift.

Question 58:
Which is true regarding X-rays?

A) X-rays do not pass through denser materials like bone and that's why they show up as white on the X-ray film.
B) X-rays pass through bone but not skin and soft tissue, and that's why bones show up white on the X-ray film.
C) X-rays don't ionise cells and thus are safe.
D) Gamma rays are safer than X-rays.

Question 59:
Rearrange $\frac{(16x+11)}{(4x+5)} = 4y^2 + 2$ to make x the subject

A) $x = \frac{20y^2-1}{[16-4(4y^2+2)]}$
B) $= \frac{20y^2-8}{[16-6(4y^2+2)]}$
C) $= \frac{6y^2-1}{[16-4(4y^2+2)]}$
D) $= \frac{21y^2-1}{[16-4(2y^2+2)]}$
E) $= \frac{7y^2-1}{[6-14(6+7)]}$

Question 60:
If $(3p + 5)^2 = 24p + 49$, calculate p.

A) -5 or -9 B) -3 or -6 C) -4 or 6 D) -6 or 4 E) 4 or -2

END OF PAPER

ANSWERS

ANSWER KEY

PAPER A				PAPER B			
Section 1	Section 2	Section 3	Section 4	Section 1	Section 2	Section 3	Section 4
1 C	23 A	41 E	53 B	1 A	23 D	41 E	53 A
2 D	24 E	42 D	54 D	2 C	24 E	42 A	54 D
3 B	25 D	43 B	55 B	3 C	25 E	43 D	55 D
4 D	26 B	44 E	56 C	4 D	26 D	44 A	56 C
5 D	27 D	45 D	57 A	5 D	27 A	45 D	57 D
6 B	28 D	46 C	58 C	6 B	28 C	46 A	58 D
7 A	29 A	47 B	59 B	7 D	29 A	47 B	59 C
8 D	30 F	48 A	60 C	8 C	30 E	48 C	60 E
9 C	31 F	49 E		9 B	31 D	49 A	
10 E	32 A	50 D		10 A	32 A	50 D	
11 E	33 C	51 E		11 E	33 D	51 C	
12 D	34 C	52 A		12 D	34 D	52 B	
13 E	35 D			13 A	35 B		
14 A	36 B			14 D	36 A		
15 D	37 A			15 E	37 E		
16 B	38 D			16 B	38 D		
17 C	39 D			17 A	39 F		
18 B	40 A			18 B	40 F		
19 D				19 E			
20 E				20 E			
21 B				21 D			
22 D				22 A			

PAPER C				PAPER D			
Section 1	Section 2	Section 3	Section 4	Section 1	Section 2	Section 3	Section 4
1 D	23 C	41 C	53 B	1 B	23 E	41 C	53 B
2 D	24 C	42 E	54 C	2 D	24 B	42 E	54 B
3 B	25 C	43 A	55 B	3 E	25 F	43 F	55 E
4 B	26 D	44 E	56 C	4 C	26 E	44 F	56 D
5 B	27 B	45 E	57 B	5 C	27 D	45 G	57 B
6 C	28 E	46 D	58 C	6 E	28 B	46 F	58 A
7 D	29 D	47 C	59 C	7 E	29 E	47 A	59 D
8 D	30 F	48 F	60 E	8 D	30 D	48 C	60 E
9 D	31 D	49 A		9 D	31 B	49 B	
10 C	32 C	50 C		10 C	32 B	50 D	
11 D	33 E	51 C		11 C	33 D	51 B	
12 E	34 E	52 E		12 B	34 D	52 E	
13 A	35 C			13 C	35 A		
14 E	36 C			14 E	36 C		
15 E	37 A			15 C	37 F		
16 E	38 E			16 B	38 H		
17 C	39 A			17 D	39 C		
18 D	40 A			18 D	40 H		
19 C				19 C			
20 B				20 B			
21 C				21 C			
22 E				22 A			

PAPER E

Section 1		Section 2		Section 3		Section 4	
1	B	**23**	F	**41**	E	**53**	D
2	B	**24**	D	**42**	F	**54**	A
3	B	**25**	A	**43**	F	**55**	C
4	D	**26**	C	**44**	B	**56**	D
5	B	**27**	E	**45**	E	**57**	B
6	D	**28**	F	**46**	B	**58**	C
7	C	**29**	E	**47**	D	**59**	E
8	B	**30**	B	**48**	D	**60**	B
9	E	**31**	B	**49**	D		
10	A	**32**	F	**50**	D		
11	C	**33**	E	**51**	E		
12	B	**34**	B	**52**	E		
13	C	**35**	A				
14	E	**36**	I				
15	D	**37**	C				
16	A	**38**	B				
17	D	**39**	D				
18	E	**40**	A				
19	D						
20	B/E						
21	D						
22	E						

PAPER F

Section 1		Section 2		Section 3		Section 4	
1	D	**23**	G	**41**	A	**53**	F
2	A	**24**	E	**42**	C	**54**	D
3	C	**25**	C	**43**	A	**55**	A
4	D	**26**	C	**44**	C	**56**	B
5	B	**27**	C	**45**	H	**57**	B
6	E	**28**	D	**46**	B	**58**	C
7	A	**29**	E	**47**	B	**59**	A
8	E	**30**	B	**48**	G	**60**	B
9	B	**31**	C	**49**	A		
10	D	**32**	D	**50**	B		
11	D	**33**	C	**51**	E		
12	B	**34**	C	**52**	B		
13	A	**35**	A				
14	E	**36**	B				
15	D	**37**	C				
16	B	**38**	B				
17	C	**39**	F				
18	B	**40**	E				
19	B						
20	E						
21	E						
22	A						

PAPER G

Section 1		Section 2		Section 3		Section 4	
1	C	**23**	B	**41**	H	**53**	D
2	E	**24**	D	**42**	B	**54**	B
3	B	**25**	E	**43**	A	**55**	B
4	D	**26**	A	**44**	F	**56**	B
5	B	**27**	D	**45**	E	**57**	B
6	E	**28**	A	**46**	A	**58**	E
7	C	**29**	B	**47**	C	**59**	B
8	E	**30**	D	**48**	D	**60**	C
9	E	**31**	D	**49**	A		
10	C	**32**	A	**50**	A		
11	B	**33**	A	**51**	B		
12	A	**34**	A	**52**	B		
13	B	**35**	C				
14	A	**36**	A				
15	B	**37**	F				
16	D	**38**	F				
17	B	**39**	E				
18	C	**40**	D				
19	E						
20	C						
21	E						
22	B						

PAPER H

Section 1		Section 2		Section 3		Section 4	
1	A	**23**	A	**41**	C	**53**	B
2	C	**24**	D	**42**	A	**54**	B
3	E	**25**	E	**43**	B	**55**	B
4	D	**26**	H	**44**	A	**56**	A
5	D	**27**	A	**45**	A	**57**	A
6	E	**28**	F	**46**	A	**58**	A
7	E	**29**	C	**47**	A	**59**	A
8	A	**30**	B	**48**	F	**60**	D
9	C	**31**	A	**49**	E		
10	D	**32**	D	**50**	D		
11	B	**33**	B	**51**	H		
12	D	**34**	A	**52**	B		
13	A	**35**	F				
14	B	**36**	E				
15	C	**37**	B				
16	B	**38**	C				
17	A	**39**	F				
18	E	**40**	E				
19	C						
20	C						
21	D						
22	A						

Mock Paper A Answers

Question 1: C

The simplest solution is to calculate the total area at the start as 20 x 20 = 400cm^2. Then recognise that with every fold the area will be reduced by half therefore the area will decrease as follows: 400, 200, 100, 50, 25, 12.5 – requiring a total of 5 folds.

Question 2: D

This is the only correct as it is the only statement that doesn't categorically state a fact that was discussed in conditional tense in the paragraph.

Question 3: B

Off the 50% carrying the parasite 20% are symptomatic. Therefore 0.5 x 0.2 = 10% of the total population are infected and symptomatic. Of which 0.1 x 0.9 = 9% are male.

Question 4: D

The most important part of the question to note is the figure of 30% reduction during sale time. Although A and B are possible the question asks specifically about cost. Therefore, it is only worth waiting for the sale period if the sterling to euro exchange rate does not depreciate more than the magnitude of the sale. As such solution D is the only correct answer as it describes anticipating a loss in sterling value less than 30% against the euro.

Question 5: D

Begin by calculating the number of childminders that can be hired for a 24-hour period as 24 x 8.5 = 204. Therefore, a total of 4 childminders can be hired continually for 24 hours with £184 left over – as the question states the hire has to be for a whole 24-hour period and therefore the remainder £184 cannot be used. As such D is the correct answer of 4 x 4 = 16.

Question 6: B

The simplest way to approach this question is to recognise that there is a difference of £1.50 between peak and off-peak prices for all individuals except students. The total savings can therefore be calculated as (3 + 5 + 1) x 1.5 = 9 x 1.5 = 13.5.

Question 7: A

Karen is a musician, so she must play an instrument, but we do not know how many instruments she plays. Although all oboe players are musicians, it does not mean all musician play the oboe. Similarly, oboes and pianos are instruments, but they are not the only instruments. So, statements b and c are incorrect. Karen is a musician but that merely means that she plays an instrument, we do not know if it is the oboe. So, statement d is incorrect.

Question 8: D

Answers A and B are simply incorrect as the measurement taken is a percentage increase (/decrease) which will normalise baseline diameters therefore allowing for comparison over multiple time points. You should be aware from your studies that ultrasound is an invaluable technique in distinguishing between adjacent tissue types. Any methodology is repeatable if it is correctly chronicled and followed therefore leaving the correct answer of D.

Question 9: C

If both the flight and travel from the airport are delayed this will be the longest the journey could possible take – producing a total journey time of 20 + 15 + 150 + 20 + 25 = 230 minutes or 3 hours 50 minutes. Therefore given all possible eventualities, to arrive at 5pm, boarding should begin at 13.10pm. Answer D is incorrect as a delayed plan would add 20 minutes to the journey whilst the transport to the meeting at the other end takes a minimum of 15 minutes – even if Megan could teleport instantaneously from the airport to the meeting she would be 5 minutes later than if there wasn't a plane delay.

Question 10: E

This is almost a trick question and simply an application of exponential decay. Recall that an exponential decay is asymptotic to 0 as no matter how small the volume within the cask becomes, only half of it is ever removed. It could be argued that this process cannot continue once a single molecule of whiskey is left – and when splitting that single molecule in half it is no longer whiskey. However, the question does not ask "how long till all the whiskey is gone" but rather "how many minutes will it take for the entire cask to be emptied" and therefore the process can continue infinitely – even if the only thing left in the cask is a collection of quarks … or half that.

Question 11: E

With these questions it is important to only consider information displayed in the graph and not involve any assumptions provided by your prior knowledge. Therefore, this question is questioning your ability to consider correlation as opposed to causation. The graph simply shows that waist size and BMI are positively correlated with one another and that is it. The nature of a scatter plot does not allow you to deduce which of the variables (if any) drives the result observed in the dependent variable. However, the fact that they are correlated is an important result and therefore D is also incorrect.

Question 12: D

A sky view of the arrangement leads to:

C	A	B	*or*	A	C	B
D		E			D	E

In both, D is to the left of E, thus is the only correct answer.

Question 13: E

The question can be expressed as (40 x 30) – x(50 x 30) = 200 = 1,200 – x1,500. Therefore x = 2/3.

Question 14: A

As the largest digit on the number pad is 9, even if 9 was pressed for an infinitely long time the entered code would still average out at no larger than 9. Therefore, it would be impossible to achieve a reference number larger than 9. Indeed, this is an extremely insecure safe but not for the reason described in B (for if the same incorrect number was pressed indefinitely it would never average out as the correct one) but rather because the safe could in theory be opened with a single digit.

Question 15: D

A is incorrect as it ignores the section of the text that states the evolution of resistant strains is driven by the presence of antibiotics themselves. The text states that the rate of bacterial reproduction is a large contributing factor and therefore not wholly responsible – hence B is incorrect. Since this is just one example (and only the information in the text should be considered for these questions) for C to make such a general statement is complete unjustified.

Question 16: B

The fastest way to solve this question is to calculate the quantity of cheese per portion as 200/10 = 20. Which for 350 people would require 350 x 20 = 7000g or 7kg.

Question 17: C

Calculate the calorific content of 12 portions as 12 x 300 = 3,600kcal. As this represents 120%, evaluate what the initial amount would be as (3,600/120) x100 = 3,000kcal.

Question 18: B

Begin by calculating the initial weight of all the ingredients in the Bolognese sauce which comes to a total of 3.05kg. Therefore when cooking for 10 people 3.05 x 4 = 12.2kg of pasta should be used. Which in turn means for 30 people 3 x 12.2 = 36.6kg should be used.

Question 19: D

Calculate the new weight of ingredients in the Bolognese sauce excluding garlic and pancetta which produces a total of 2.8kg. Note that onions represent 0.3kg per 10 people and as such the ratio can be represented as 0.3/2.8 or alternatively dividing top and bottom by 0.3 → 1/9.3

Question 20: E

Begin with calculating total preparation time as 25 x 4 = 100 mins. The fact that Simon can only cook 8 portions at a time is somewhat a red herring as it doesn't impact the calculation. Total cooking time can be calculated as a further 25 x 8 = 200 mins. Producing a total time of 300mins or 5 hours.

Question 21: B

This is a general knowledge question, a quick google search tells you that the answer is Miguel de Cervantes

Question 22: D

General knowledge question

Question 23: A

An organ is defined as comprising multiple tissue types. As blood and skeletal muscle are themselves tissues they cannot be classified as organs.

Question 24: E

This question is best considered in terms of the aerobic respiration equation. With that in mind it becomes apparent that increased forward drive through the reaction will produce large amounts of water and CO_2 whilst demanding an increased supply of O_2. Further from this equation we realise that aerobic respiration produces large amounts of heat, and as such it is expected – in the interest of thermoregulation – that the body will both perspire and vasodilate in attempt to increase heat loss. Therefore, E is the correct answer.

Question 25: D

Recall that the nephron is the smallest functional unit of the kidney. The question therefore is asking you what is the smallest basic functional unit of striated muscle? To which the answer is the sarcomere. Note that a myofibril is a collection of many sarcomeres and is therefore not the correct answer.

Question 26: B

Insulin is a polypeptide hormone released by the pancreas in response to elevated plasma glucose levels. Therefore, it can be expected that plasma glucose concentration will be proportional to the concentration of insulin in the blood. Furthermore, recall that glucagon also released by the pancreas mobilises glucose stores. Therefore, the greatest concentration of plasma glucose would be expected at the time when glucagon is highest during a period of elevated insulin.

Question 27: D

Answers a and c are both nonsense and can be eliminated straight away. You will know from your study of the immune system that it is plasma B cells that produce antibodies and that plasma T cells do not exist. Also recall that an immune response can be mounted as quickly as within a fortnight which leaves the only correct answer d. The passage states that only once blood types are mixed is the immune response initiated, therefore answer d provides an explanation as to how this happens but also why the first-born child is unaffected.

Question 28: D

An organ consists of many cell types which once differentiated are committed to that single cell line. Therefore, a totipotent stem cell is required to produce the multiple cell types required. In order to ensure that the organ is an exact genetic match, stem cells from the individual in question must be used. Unless that individual is an embryo, adult stem cells must be used

Question 29: A

DNA consists of 4 bases: adenine, guanine, thymine and cysteine. The sugar backbone consists of deoxyribose, hence the name DNA. DNA is found in the cytoplasm of prokaryotes

Question 30: F

Mitochondria are responsible for energy production by ATP synthesis. Animal cells do not have a cell wall, only a cell membrane. The endoplasmic reticulum is important in protein synthesis, as this is where the proteins are assembled.

Question 31: F

If you aren't studying A-level biology, this question may stretch you. However, it is possible to reach an answer by process of elimination. Mitochondria are the 'powerhouse' of the cell in aerobic respiration, responsible for cell energy production rather than DNA replication or protein synthesis. As energy producers they are required in muscle cells in large numbers, and in sperm cells to drive the tail responsible for movement. They are enveloped by a double membrane, possibly because they started out as independent prokaryotes engulfed by eukaryotic cells.

Question 32: A

The majority of bacteria are commensals and don't lead to disease.

Question 33: C

Bacteria carry genetic information on plasmids and not in nuclei like animal cells. They don't need meiosis for replication, as they do not require gametes. Bacterial genomes consist of DNA, just like animal cells.

Question 34: C

Active transport requires a transport protein and ATP, as work is being done against an electrochemical gradient. Unlike diffusion, the relative concentrations of the materials being transported aren't important.

Question 35: D

Meiosis produces haploid gametes. This allows for fusion of 2 gametes to reach a full diploid set of chromosomes again in the zygote.

Question 36: B

Mendelian inheritance separates traits into dominant or recessive. It applies to all sexually reproducing organisms. Don't get confused by statement C – the offspring of 2 heterozygotes has a 25% chance of expressing a recessive trait, but it will be homozygous recessive.

Question 37: A

Hormones are released into the bloodstream and act on receptors in different organs in order to cause relatively slow changes to the body's physiology. Hormones frequently interact with the nervous system, e.g. Adrenaline and Insulin, however, they don't directly cause muscles to contract. Almost all hormones are synthesised.

Question 38 D

Neuronal signalling can happen via direct electrical stimulation of nerves or via chemical stimulation of synapses which produces a current that travels along the nerves. Electrical synapses are very rare in mammals, the majority of mammalian synapses are chemical.

Question 39: D

Remember that pH changes cause changes in electrical charge on proteins (= polypeptides) that could interfere with protein – protein interactions. Whilst the other statements are all correct to a certain extent, they are the downstream effects of what would happen if enzymes (which are also proteins) didn't work.

Question 40: A

The bacterial cell wall is made up of murein and protects the bacterium from the external environment, in particular from osmotic stresses, and is important in most bacteria.

Question 41: E

Recall that pH is a logarithmic scale of proton concentration and therefore will have the largest effect on hydrogen bonding.

Question 42: D

Isotopes of an element all contain the same number of protons but a different number of neutrons. As atomic number refers solely to the number of protons it will not change. However as mass number is the sum of atomic number and neutron number – it would be expected to change. If an isotope contains one extra proton, then assuming the charge of that isotope is 0, then it must also contain one extra electron. Chemical properties are the same for all isotopes. Therefore, the correct answer is D.

Question 43: B

The transition metals are the most abundant catalysts – presumably due to their ability to achieve a variable number of stable states. Therefore, the correct answer is the d-block elements.

Question 44: E

Begin by writing down the balanced equation that describes the reaction of francium with water: $2Fr + 2H_2O \rightarrow 2FrOH + H_2$. Next calculate the moles of francium entering the reaction as 1338/223 = 6. We therefore know from the stoichiometry of the equation that this reaction will produce 3 moles of hydrogen. Recall that 1 mole of gas at room temperature and pressure occupies $24dm^3$. Therefore, the hydrogen produced in this reaction will occupy 3 x 24 = $72dm^3$.

Question 45: D

The simplest way to approach this type of question is to assume that there are 10 atoms within the compound. In this case that produces the following result: $C_3H_4F_2Cl$. Next look to see if any of the subscript numbers are divisible by a common factor. Also, if there are any decimals, multiply up by a common factor until only integers are present. In this case the correct answer is achieved straight away.

Question 46: C

This question requires you to have a correct answer from the previous question, although these questions are unfair in the fact that this current question cannot be answered without success in the first part – there are always one or two of these per paper. Simply calculate the Mr of your empirical formula: 113.5. And then divide 340.5 by this: 340.5/113.5 = 3. Therefore, multiply your empirical formula up by a factor of 3.

Question 47: B

The calculation in this question is simple: concentration = mass/volume, what this question is really testing is the manipulation of unorthodox units. Begin by noting the use of g/dL in the final answers and therefore begin by converting the quantities in the question into these units. 1.2×10^{10} kg = 1.2×10^{13} grams and with 10 decilitres in a litre, 4×10^{12} L = 4×10^{13} dL. $\frac{(1.2 \times 10^{13})}{(4 \times 10^{13})} = 3 \times 10^{-1}$ g/dL.

Question 48: A

A catalyst is not essential for the progression of a chemical reaction, it only acts to lower the activation energy and therefore increase the likelihood and rate of reaction.

Question 49: E

Cationic surfactants represent a class of molecule that demonstrates both hydrophilic and hydrophobic domains. This allows it to act as an emulsifying agent which is particularly useful in the disruption of grease or lipid deposits. Therefore, cationic surfactants have applications in all the products listed.

Question 50: D

Different isotopes are differentiated by the number of neutrons in the core. This gives them different molecular weights and different chemical properties with regards to stability. The number of protons defines each element, and the number of electrons its charge.

Question 51: E

A displacement reaction occurs when a more reactive element displaces a less reactive element in its compound. All 4 reactions are examples of displacement reactions as a less reactive element is being replaced by a more reactive one.

Question 52: A

There needs to be 3Ca, 12H, 14O and 2P on each side. Only option A satisfies this.

Question 53: B

Let tail = T, body and legs = B and head = H.

As described in the question H = T + 0.5B and B = T + H. We have already been told that T = 30Kg.

Therefore, substitute the second equation into the first as H = 30 + 0.5(30 + H).

Re-arranging reveals that -0.5H = 45Kg and therefore the weight of the head is 90Kg, the body and legs 120Kg and as we were told the tail weighs 30Kg. Thus, giving a total weight of 240Kg

Question 54: D

Recall that kinetic energy can be calculated as $E = 0.5mv^2$. Therefore, if mass remains constant it is the v^2 term that must be reduced to a sixteenth. In other words, $v^2 = 1/16$ and therefore the correct velocity is $1/4x$.

Question 55: B

Recall that V = E/Q; therefore, when substituting SI units into these equation it is discovered that $V = J/C = JC^{-1}$.

Question 56: C

Recall that voltmeters are always connected in parallel – and so that they don't draw any current from the circuit have an infinite resistance. Ammeters on the other hand are connected in series and therefore must not perturb the flow of given, meaning they have zero resistance.

Question 57: A

Much of the information in this question is not needed and is simply put there to distract you. This question can be most quickly solved using the equation F=ma or force = mass x acceleration. As object A is the only things moving in this scenario it is the only source of energy to be considered. Its mass will be the same before and after the collision and so we need only calculate the magnitude of retardation. Given as $(15 - 3)/0.5 = 24ms^{-2}$. Therefore, when plugging into the first equation we realise that F = 12 x 24 = 288N of force dissipated. Alternatively, this question could be solved by calculating the rate of change of momentum.

Question 58: C

Note the atomic masses and numbers in the equation. Whilst the atomic mass has remained constant the atomic number has increased by one and hence the element has changed. The only explanation for this is that a neutron has turned into a proton (and an electron which is represented by *x*). Therefore, the correct answer is C – beta radioactive decay.

Question 59: B

Begin by calculating the velocity of the wave as speed = wavelength x frequency = 3 x 20 = 60km/s. Which in a time period of one hour (3600s) would equate to a total distance of 60 x 3600 = 216,000km.

Question 60: C

The numerator of the fraction consists of 3 distinct terms or 3 distinct dimensions. As all other functions within the equation are constants one would consider this the volume of a complex 3D shape.

END OF PAPER

Mock Paper B Answers

Question 1: A

If society disagree that vaccinations should be compulsory, then they will not fund them. So, statement A is correct. It attacks the conclusion. Statement b - society does not necessarily mean local so this does not address the argument. Statement c strengthens, not weakens, the argument for vaccinations. Statement d – the wants of healthcare workers do not affect whether vaccinations are necessary.

Question 2: C

Start by calculating the area of wall that may be painted per tin of paint as 10 x 5 = 50m^2. Therefore, to paint the whole area 1050/50 = 21 tins of paint are required per coat. As such to complete 3 coats it will cost Josh 3 x 21 x 4.99 = 314.37.

Question 3: C

A is a correct assumption as procession is a function of rotational motion. B is a necessary assumption or rather inference of the first sentence. The second sentence only says that an asterism can be used, not that it is the only possible method. Nothing is mentioned of navigating the Southern Hemisphere and therefore C is not a valid assumption.

Question 4: D

Recognise that "bank hours" refers only to hours that the bank is open – which Mon to Fri is 8 hours whereas it is only 6 hours on a Saturday. Although John needs the money by 8pm the bank closes at 5 and that 3 hours difference cannot be used. Hence working backwards John will need 8 hours on the Tuesday, 8 hours on the Monday, Sunday is closed, 6 hours on the Saturday, 8 hours on Friday and 8 hours on Thursday and 4 hours on the Wednesday. With a closing time of 5pm, the latest John can cash the cheque on Wednesday is 1pm.

Question 5: D

First thing to recognise here of course is that individual diamonds can be combined to form larger diamonds with the 5 x 5 diamond the biggest of them all. To avoid counting them all and risking losing count, instead deduced the number of triangles per corner and per side; then multiply up by 4.

Question 6: B

Let my current age = m and my brother's current age = g. The first section of this question can therefore be expressed as m + 4 = 1/3(g + 1) whereas the second half can be represented as 2(m + 20) = g + 20. Therefore, this problem can be solved as simultaneous equations. Rearranged the second equation reads m = 1/2g - 10; when substituted into the first equation we form 1/2g – 10 + 4 = 1/3(g + 1). Expand and simplify to 1/2g – 6 = 1/3g + 1/3 → 1/6g = $6\frac{1}{3}$ which therefore means my brother's current age = $6\frac{1}{3}$ / (1/6) = 114/3 = 38. Which means that my current age = 1/2(38) – 10 = 9.

Question 7: D

A is categorically wrong as the first two paragraphs discuss how aneurysms produce inflammation which in turn blunts endothelial NO action. B is incorrect as it states aneurysms directly promote CVD, this is not a direct process. It is the blunted NO which directly produces the CVD. C can be ignored as nowhere are aneurysms categorised like this. E is incorrect as the text states that aneurysms reduce NO which will reduce vasodilatation, thus increasing basal vasoconstriction and thus reducing blood flow. Leaving the correct answer of D which is of course true as observations are not transferable between species until tested scientifically.

Question 8: C

Any statement which refers to national or global figures is instantly incorrect as the text does not mention any statistical analysis has taken place. In order to produce national statistics from a small sample size such as this requires statistical analysis. Whilst E could possibly be true it cannot be stated as there are so many possibilities – perhaps the time of the survey was during rush hour in which case the majority of the traffic would have been travelling in the same direction anyway to reach an industrialised area.

Question 9: B

The runners aren't apart at a constant distance; they get further apart as they run. Xavier and Yolanda are less than 20m apart at the time William finishes. Each runner beats the next runner by the same distance, so they must have the same difference between speeds. When William finishes at 100m and Xavier is at 80m. When Xavier crosses the finish line then Yolanda is at 80m. We need to know where Yolanda is when Xavier is at 80m. William's speed = distance/time = 100/T. Xavier's speed = 80/T. So, Xavier has 80% of William's speed. This makes Yolanda's speed 80% of Xavier's and 64% (80% x 80% = 64%) of William's. So, when William is at 64m when William finishes. 100m - 64m = 36m, thus William beats Yolanda by 36m.

Question 10: A

This question can be solved quickly if you first realise that there is no need to calculate both volumes and subtract the larger from the smaller, instead only convert the television dimensions into metres and then calculate 60% of that.

Question 11: E

From the information provided all the flaws listed are valid since David's main point is that he has chosen the cheapest. A could be true as there is an additional cost of £3 for staying at Whitmore, therefore if the vehicle they are using achieves sufficient miles per gallon then travelling the extra few miles could cost less than £3 in terms of petrol. B again is possible which would argue against it being cheap, as would D. And if C is true then David's argument is flawed altogether.

Question 12: D

C is irrelevant as nowhere does the passage mention standards of modern medical practice. A may be incorrect as nowhere does the article explicitly say that animal testing is the only accepted method of drug approval. B categorically conflicts with the first sentence of the second paragraph.

Question 13: A

Begin by converting all the quantities into terms of items as that is the terminology used on the graph axis. Therefore 12 rugby balls = 6 items and 120 tennis balls = 24 items. Reading from the graph reveals their respective prices as £9 and £5. Therefore, the total cost of products in the order is (6 x 9) + (24 x 5) = 174. Since this is significantly more than £100 the delivery charge is waived.

Question 14: D

Calculate the cost of 10 of everything as (2 x 5) x (10 x 7) x (5 x 9) = £125. Recall that delivery charge is waived at £100 and this therefore a trick question and no delivery charge is applied anyway.

Question 15: E

Tennis balls are sold in the largest pack and so they must be considered. Begin by dividing 1000/5 using the value from the first column = 200. As this is above the range 0 -99 look up the item value in the 100 -499 range where a £1 discount is applied per item. Therefore, in actually fact 1000/4 = 250 items can be purchased which equates to a total of 250 x 5 = 1250 balls.

Question 16: B

Recognise that 120% profit is equivalent to 220% of the original price. In which case the initial purchase price = (1,320/220) x 100 = £600.

Question 17: A

Note that here the question uses the term item and therefore simply read the costs directly off the graph giving a total order cost of (2 x 2000) + (4 x 2000) + (6 x 2000) = 24,000. Recall though that he only pays tax on the amount over £12,000 which in this case is £12,000. Therefore, he pays 12,000/4 = £3,000 tax.

Question 18: B

Lucy must live between Vicky and Shannon. Lucy is Vicky's neighbour, so Shannon cannot have a red door. Vicky lives next to someone with a red door, so Lucy must have the red door. This leaves Shannon with the blue door and Lucy with the white. The green door is across the road and so does not belong to any of them.

Question 19: E

First calculate an average complete one-way journey time as 40 + 5 + 5 = 50 minutes. Deducting his breaks, he works a total of 7 hours 20 or 440 minutes. Since the first train is already loaded his first run will only take 45 minutes leaving 395 minutes to complete his working day. 395/50 = 7 remainder 45. Note that 45 minutes is not enough to fully unload the train, but it is enough to load the train and drive the distance. Therefore, the driver will complete a total of 9 journeys equalling a distance of 198 miles.

Question 20: E

A is not actually a valid assumption as we do not know what proposal conservationists might be bringing to the local councils, they have only expressed their concern. They may well be bringing a proposal to ask for funding to rehome all the species in the affected environment. B is essential to the final paragraph whilst C must be assumed otherwise the councils would not be presenting these proposals at all.

Question 21: D

General knowledge question

Question 22: A

General knowledge question

Question 23: D

As the question states that GLUT2 is ATP independent then answer A) active transport is instantly incorrect as it is ATP dependent. Osmosis is applicable only to water molecules and is therefore incorrect. Exocytosis refers to the movement of molecules out of a cell and is therefore incorrect. Simple diffusion is incorrect as the question states that GLUT2 is essential for the process. This leaves the correct answer of facilitated diffusion.

Question 24: E

Firstly, recall that endocytosis is a process of molecular transport into cells that result in vesicular formation. This question requires you to realise the special case of this which is phagocytosis – conducted by white blood cells in the ingestion of pathogens.

Question 25: E

All of the above statements are true of the Calvin cycle with regards to the Krebs cycle. As the main driver of photosynthesis, we know that the Calvin cycle requires both CO_2 and light in order to conduct ATP dependent reactions. As opposed to the Krebs cycle in man however, the Calvin cycle adopts the use of NADPH as the intermediate in electron transport.

Question 26: D

Option D is one of only 2 graphs that demonstrate a quadratic relationship with the peak enzyme activity correctly placed – pepsin from the stomach close to pH 1, and trypsin secreted by the pancreas and therefore alkaline around pH 13. The curves traced in option c however are far too broad over the pH range to represent enzyme activity. As the pH scale is logarithmic, even a change of 1 or 0.5 can be devastating to enzyme activity.

Question 27: A

This question was taken directly from the IMAT syllabus where many examples are listed for different principles. Reading the IMAT syllabus and highlighting these is a very good idea as well as learning the definitions listed.

Question 28: C

Sexual reproduction relies on formation of gametes during **meiosis**. Mitosis doesn't produce genetically distinct cells. Mitosis is, however, the basis for tissue growth.

Question 29: A

A mutation is a permanent change in the nucleotide sequence of DNA. Whilst mutations may lead to changes in organelles and chromosomes, or even be harmful, they are strictly defined as permanent changes to the DNA or RNA sequence.

Question 30: E

Mutations are fairly common, but in the vast majority of cases do not have any impact on phenotype due to the redundancy of the genome. Sometimes they can confer selective advantages and allow organisms to survive better (i.e. evolve by natural selection), or they can lead to cancers as cells start dividing uncontrollably.

Question 31: D

Antibodies represent a pivotal molecule of the immune system. They provide very pointed and selective targeting of pathogens and toxins without causing damage to the body's own cells.

Question 32: A

Kidneys are not involved in digestion, but do filter the blood of waste products. Glucose is found in high concentrations in the urine of diabetics, who cannot absorb it without working insulin.

Question 33: D

Hormones are slower acting than nerves and act for a longer time. Hormones also act in a more general way. Adrenaline is also a hormone released into the body causing the fight-or-flight response. Although it is quick acting, it still lasts for a longer time than a nervous response, as you can still feel its effects for a time after the response, e.g. shaking hands.

Question 34: D

Homeostasis is about minimising changes to the internal environment by modulating both input and output.

Question 35: B

There is less energy and biomass each time you move up a trophic level. Only 10% of consumed energy is transferred to the next trophic level, so only one tenth of the previous biomass can be sustained in the next trophic level up.

Question 36: A

In asexual reproduction, there is no fusion of gametes as the single parent cell divides. There is therefore no mixing of chromosomes and, as a result, no genetic variation.

Question 37: E

The image is first formed on the retina which conveys it to the brain via a sensory nerve. The brain then sends an impulse to the muscle via a motor neuron.

Question 38: D

Blood from the kidney returns to the heart via the renal (kidney-related) vein, which drains into the inferior vena cava. The blood then passes through the pulmonary vasculature (veins carry blood to the heart, arteries away from the heart) before going into the aorta and eventually the hepatic (liver-related) artery.

Question 39: F

Clones are genetically identical by definition, and a large number of them could conceivably reduce the gene pool of a population. In adult cell cloning, the genetic material of an egg is replaced with the genetic material of an adult cell. Cloning is possible for all DNA based life forms, including plants and other types of animals.

Question 40: F

Gene varieties cause intraspecies variation, e.g. different eye colours. If mutations confer a selective advantage, those individuals with the mutation will survive to reproduce and grow in numbers. Genetic variation is caused by mixing of parent genomes and mutations. Species with similar characteristics often do have similar genes.

Question 41: E

In order to answer this question you must recall that anaerobic respiration in humans produces only lactate and energy, whilst in yeast the anaerobic respiratory process yields a molecule of ethanol and CO_2 per glucose molecule. Therefore, there will be 0 mol of CO_2 produced in the human cell culture and you need only work out the moles of CO_2 produced by the yeast cell culture to calculate the difference. There is a total of 5.76/0.18 = 32 mol of glucose, of which half is supplied to the yeast cell culture. With a stoichiometric ratio of 1:1 in the anaerobic respiration equation a total of 16 mol of CO_2 will be produced.

Question 42: A

Initially the electron configuration of Mg is 2,8,2. In binding to two chlorine atoms it is effectively ionised to Mg^{2+} and it loses two electrons to leave a complete outer shell and thus the correct answer is 2,8.

Question 43: D

The first thing to note in this trace is that the m/z axis has been cut short. From looking up the mass of calcium in the periodic table one would expect to see the x axis centred around 40. However here the trace is only displaying those isotopes with valence 2 (z= 2) hence the values are half the size. Therefore (from the periodic table) when dividing the most abundant isotope of chromium by two, 52/2 = 26, we confirm that the outlier bar on the right is indeed the contaminant. Therefore, to calculate the actual abundance of Mr 40 calcium ignore the chromium like so: 55/95 = 11/19.

Question 44: A

Begin by converting the total weight of arsenic into grams like so $15 \times 10^6 = 1.5 \times 10^7$. Then divide by the Mr of arsenic which is 75 (2sf) giving 2×10^5. Don't forget that the sample is at worst 80% pure. Therefore, there will be a minimum of $(2 \times 10^5) \times 0.8 = 1.4 \times 10^5$ moles of pure arsenic.

Question 45: D

Recall that average atomic mass is calculated as the sum of (isotope mass x relative abundance). Therefore $28 = (26 \times 0.6) + (30 \times 0.3) + 0.1x$. Rearranging this equation reveals that $0.1x = 3.4$ and that the mystery isotope therefore has an atomic mass of 34.

Question 46: A

First recall that when a group 2 metal is reacted with steam a metal oxide is formed and therefore the following chemical equation can be drawn: $Mg + H_2O_{(g)} \rightarrow MgO + H_2$. Note the stoichiometric ratio which is simply 1. Next calculate that there is 72/24 = 3 mol of hydrogen produced. Therefore, assuming that there is 3 mol of all other reactants and the reaction is complete one would expect 3 x 24.3 = 72.9g of magnesium and 3 x 18 = 54g of steam. This is indeed the case and therefore the reaction is complete.

Question 47: B

The reducing agent is the species which is itself reduced in this instance from looking at the oxidation states we can see that that species is S^{2-}. As after the reaction has taken place it has an oxidation state of +6 which would require a loss of negative charge i.e. electrons.

Question 48: C

The highly stable bonds between carbon atoms, and between carbon and hydrogen atoms renders alkanes relatively unreactive. This is important to note as it highlights the major difference between alkanes and alkenes.

Question 49: A

To balance the equation there needs to be 9Ag, 9N, $9O_3$, 9K, 3P on each side. Only option A satisfies this.

Question 50: D
A more reactive halogen can displace a less reactive halogen. Thus, chlorine can displace bromine and iodine from an aqueous solution of its salts, and fluorine can replace chlorine. The trend is the opposite for alkali metals, where reactivity increases down the group as electrons are further from the core and easier to lose.

Question 51: C
$2Mg + O_2 = 2MgO$; so, 2 x 24 = 48 and 2 x (24 + 16) = 80; so, 48 g of magnesium produces 80g of magnesium oxide; so 1g of magnesium produces 1g x 80g/48g = 1.666g oxide; so 75g x 1.666 = 125g

Question 52: B
$H_2 + 2OH^- \rightarrow 2H_2O + e^-$. Thus, the hydrogen loses electrons i.e. is oxidised.

Question 53: A
Recall that current = charge/time. The question provides both charge and time in the correct units and so the calculation is relatively simple with no unit conversions required. Therefore current = 5/15 = 1/3 = 0.33A. As the question states that the balloon has a negative charge it has therefore gained electrons. Given that a current is defined as a net movement of electrons, in this situation the current must be flowing into the balloon.

Question 54: D
Given that Power = IV it can be deduced that I = P/V. Recall that power given in Watts is a measure of the energy transferred per second and therefore has the alternative units Js^{-1}. When substituting these units into the power equation re-arranged for Amps it is revealed that $I = (Js^{-1})/V = A$.

Question 55: D
For a transformer that is 100% efficient power in must equal power out, recalling that P=IV. Therefore, the transformer has a power output of 24 x 10 = 240W which is 80% of the initial input. As such the initial power input was (240/80) x 100 = 300W.

Question 56: C
Begin by calculating the energy required to hoist the mass, this is calculated using the potential energy equation: mgh. Energy = mass x g x height = 20 x 10 x 30 = 6000N. The power output of the motor is calculated as the joules dissipated per second = 6000/20 = 300W

Question 57: D
In order to solve this problem, recall that activity = decay constant x number of remaining atoms. Therefore, the decay constant can be calculated simply as 0.36/6 = 0.06.

Question 58: D
Recall that household electricity is available in the UK at 240V. Begin by calculating the wattage that the bulb is receiving as 0.5 x 240 = 120W. Given that the energy rating of the bulb is 80W, we can assume that this bulb is only 80/120 = 66% efficient.

Question 59: C
The formula for calculating compound interest can be given as investment x (interest rate^{years}) or in short hand for this situation: $1687.5 = 500x^3$. Therefore, in order to calculate the interest rate the above formula must be rearranged to $\sqrt[3]{1687.5/500} = 1.5$ revealing an interest rate of 50%.

Question 60: E

Begin by subtracting the integral from both sides producing $x - \int_{-z}^{z} 9a - 7 = \frac{\sqrt{b^3-9st}}{13j}$. Next multiply both sides by 13j and square, rendering $[13j(x - \int_{-z}^{z} 9a - 7)]^2 = b^3 - 9st$. Finally subtract b^3 from both sides and divide by -9s leaving the correct answer: $\frac{[13j(x - \int_{-z}^{z} 9a - 7)]^2 - b^3}{-9s} = t$.

END OF PAPER

Mock Paper C Answers

Question 1: D

There are three different options for staying at the hotel. They could either pay for three single rooms for £180, one single and one double room for £165, or one four-person room for £215.

Subtracting the cleaning cost for one night would leave:
£180-(3x£12) = £144
£165-(2x£12) = £141
£215-£12 = £203

The cheapest option is one single and one double room, and they want to stay three nights, which gives £141x3 = £423.

Question 2: D

Glass one starts with 16ml squash and 80ml water. Glass two starts with 72ml squash and 24ml water. 48ml is half of 96ml so 8ml squash and 40ml water is transferred to glass two. Glass two now contains (8+72 = 80ml squash) and (24+40 = 64ml water). Glass two now has a total of 144ml and half of this is transferred to glass one. Glass one now has (40+8 = 48ml squash) and (32+40 = 72ml water). Therefore, glass one has 48ml squash and glass two has 40ml squash.

Question 3: B

B is the main conclusion of the argument. Options A and D both contribute reasons to support the main conclusion of the argument that the HPV vaccination should remain in schools. C is a counter argument, which is a reason given in opposition to the main conclusion. Option E represents a general principle behind the main argument.

Question 4: B

The speed of the bus can be calculated using the relationship: Speed $= \frac{\text{distance}}{\text{time}}$

$\frac{3\text{ km}}{0.2\text{ h}} = 15\text{ kmh}^{-1}$

The bike speed is therefore ($\frac{4}{5}$ x 15 = 12 kmh^{-1}). Considering that the bus leaves 2 minutes after the bike, it is now possible to write an expression, where d is the distance travelled when the bus overtakes the bike:

$$\frac{d\text{ km}}{12\text{ km/h}} = \frac{1}{30}\text{h} + \frac{d\text{ km}}{15\text{ km/h}}$$

This expression can be solved by multiplying each term by (12 kmh^{-1} x 15 kmh^{-1}):
15d km = 6 km +12d km
3d km = 6 km
d = 2 km

Therefore, the bus overtakes the bike after travelling 2 km.

Question 5: B

Firstly, determine who will move up to set one. Terry, Bahara, Lucy and Shiv all have attendance over 95%. Alex, Bahara and Lucy all have an average test mark over 92. Terry, Bahara, Lucy and Shiv all have less than 5% homework handed in late. Therefore, Bahara and Lucy will both move up a set. Secondly, determine who will receive a certificate. Terry, Bahara, Lucy and Shiv have absences below 4%. Alex, Bahara and Lucy have an average test mark over 89. Bahara and Shiv have at least 98% homework handed in on time. Therefore, only Bahara will receive a certificate.

Question 6: C

Firstly, construct two algebraic equations: A-18=B-25 and $A=\frac{5}{6}B$

Solve these two equations as simultaneous equations by substituting $\frac{5}{6}B$ for A in equation 1:

$\frac{5}{6}B-18=B-25$

$7=\frac{1}{6}B$

B=42

Put B=42 back into equation 2: $A= 42 \times \frac{5}{6}$

A=35

Question 7: D

I need to make 48 scones, which makes up 8 batches.
8 batches would take: 35+ 7(25+10) +25 = 305 minutes

I need to make 32 cupcakes, which makes up 4 batches.
4 batches would take: 15+ (4x20) =95 minutes

I need to make 48 cucumber sandwiches
This would take (8x5) = 40 minutes

Adding 305, 95 and 40 minutes is 440 minutes in total. 440 minutes is equivalent to 7 hours and 20 minutes. Adding 7 hours and 20 minutes to 10:45am leads to 6:05pm so I will be finished at 6:05pm.

Question 8: D

The volume of a pyramid is given by the equation:

$v=\frac{a^2h}{3}$ where v=volume, a=base and h=height

Rearrange to work out the height for each pyramid: $h=\frac{3v}{a^2}$

Pyramid	Base edge (m)	Volume (m^3)	Calculation:	Height (m)
1	3	33	$\frac{3 \times 33}{9}$	11
2	4	64	$\frac{3 \times 64}{16}$	12
3	2	8	$\frac{3 \times 8}{4}$	6
4	6	120	$\frac{3 \times 120}{36}$	10
5	2	8	$\frac{3 \times 8}{4}$	6
6	6	120	$\frac{3 \times 120}{36}$	10
7	4	64	$\frac{3 \times 64}{16}$	12

The tallest pyramid is 12m and the smallest is 6m. Subtracting the height of the tallest pyramid from the height of the smallest pyramid leaves 6m.

Question 9: D

There are 10 passengers on the tube at the final stop. At stop 5 there were twice the number of passengers on the tube so 20 passengers were at stop 5. At stop 4, there were $\frac{5}{2}$ times the number of passengers at stop 5 so 50 passengers were present at stop 4. At stop 3, there were $\frac{3}{2}$ times the number of passengers at stop 4 so 75 passengers were on the tube. At stop 2, there were $\frac{6}{5}$ times the number of passengers at stop 3 so 90 passengers were present at stop 2. Similarly, at stop 1, there were $\frac{6}{5}$ times the number of passengers at stop 2 so at the first stop 108 passengers got on the tube.

Question 10: C

The main conclusion is C. A and B both represent reasons to support the main conclusion of the argument. Option D represents an assumption that is not stated in the argument but is required to support the main conclusion that research universities should strongly support teaching. Option E is a counter argument that provides a reason to oppose the main argument.

Question 11: D

D is the main conclusion of the argument. A is a general principle of the argument, but the argument is more specific to the use of helmets rather than the wider concept of danger in sport and the responsibilities of the governing bodies to sports players. Options B and C are reasons to support the main conclusion. Option E is an intermediate conclusion, which acts as support for the next stage of the argument and as a reason to support the main conclusion.

Question 12: E

- Some students born in winter like English, Art and Music
- There is not enough information to tell whether some students born in spring like both Biology and Maths.
- We don't know what the students born in spring think about Art.
- We don't know what the students born in winter think about Biology.
- There is not enough information to know whether this is true or not.

Subject	TIME OF BIRTH		
	SPRING	AUTUMN	WINTER
English	Everyone likes	Everyone likes	Everyone likes
Biology	Some like	No one likes	
Art		Everyone likes	Some like
Music			Everyone likes
Maths	Some like		

Question 13: A

The main conclusion is option A that some works of modern art no longer constitute art. B is not an assumption made by the author as the main conclusion does not rely on *all* modern art being ugly to be valid. C is not an assumption because the argument does not rely on artists studying for decades to produce pieces of work that constitute art. This point is simply used to support the main argument. Options D and E are stated in the argument so are not assumptions. A is an assumption because it is required to be true to support the main conclusion but is not explicitly stated in the argument.

Question 14: E

Reducing the price of the sunglasses by 10% is equivalent to multiplying the price by 0.9. the price of the sunglasses is successively reduced by 10% three times and so the price on Monday is 0.9^3 the price of the sunglasses on Friday. 0.9^3 is equal to 0.729 and so the price of the sunglasses on Monday is 72.9% of the price of the sunglasses on Friday.

Question 15: E

Look at the flat cube net and note the shapes that are adjacent to each other. Sides that are joining on the net will be beside each other on the formed cube. Work through to deduce option E can be formed from the cube net shown.

Question 16: E

The information provided about the child needs to be inserted into the BMI formula: BMI=35 ÷ 1.2^2

1.2 squared is equal to 1.44 and it may be easier to work out 3500 divided by 144. The answer needs to be worked out to 3 decimal places for an answer required to 2 decimal places. The answer to 3 decimal places is 24.305 and so the BMI to 2 decimal places is 24.31.

Question 17: C

It is important that the information is inserted into the formula given for calculating the BMR of a woman rather than a man:

BMR= (10 x weight in kg) + (6.25 x height in cm) – (5 x age in years) -161

BMR = (10 x 80) + (6.25 x 170) – (5 x 32) – 161

BMR= 800 + 1062.5 -160 -161

The BMR of the woman in the question is therefore 1541.5 kcal

Question 18: D

This time, the information needs to be inserted into the formula for calculating the BMI of a man:

BMR= (10 x weight in kg) + (6.25 x height in cm) – (5 x age in years) + 5

BMR= (10 x 80) + (6.25 x 170) – (5 x 45) +5

BMR= 800 + 1062.5 -225 +5

The BMR of the man in the question is therefore 1642.5 kcal. The man does little to no exercise each week. It is therefore required to multiply 1642.5 by 1.2, which gives a daily recommended intake of 1971 kcal.

Question 19: C

It is easier to write out this calculation in the following format:

```
a b 7 –
  a b
_______
5 6 5
```

From the above subtraction it is clear that b must be equal to 2 because 7 minus 2 is equal to 5, which is the unit term of the answer. It is now possible to rewrite the calculation with 2 substituted for b:

```
a 2 7 –
  a 2
_______
5 6 5
```

From the above calculation it is possible to gauge certain facts. A must be greater than 5 because 1 is carried over to the second term:

```
a̸ ¹2 7 –
   a 2
_______
 5 6 5
```

It is now clear than a must be equal to 6 because 12 minus 6 is equal to 6, which is the tens value of the answer.

Question 20: B

The mean is the sum of all of the numbers divided by the number of terms. From the information, we know that the sum of the first 8 numbers divided by 8 is equal to 44 plus the sum of the first 8 numbers all divided by 10. An expression for this can be written like this:

$$\frac{\text{sum of 8 numbers}}{8} = y = \frac{\text{sum of 8 numbers+44}}{10}$$

Two equations can be derived from the above expression:

$10y$ = sum of 8 numbers +44
$8y$ = sum of 8 numbers

If we subtract the second equation from the first, we are left with: $2y=44 \rightarrow y=22$

The value of y and the average of both sets of numbers is therefore 22.

Question 21: C

General knowledge question

Question 22: E

General knowledge question

Question 23: C

Statement 1 is true. High temperatures and pH extremes cause a permanent alteration to the highly specific shape of the active site so that the substrate can no longer bind, and the enzyme no longer works.
Statement 2 is false. Amylase is produced in the salivary glands, pancreas, and small intestine.
Statement 3 is true.
Statement 4 is false. Bile is stored in the gall bladder, but it does travel down the bile duct to neutralise hydrochloric acid found in the stomach.
Statement 5 is true. Fructose is sweeter than glucose so smaller amounts can be used in food used in the slimming industry.

Question 24: C

The combining of food with bile and digestive enzymes occurs in the duodenum of the small intestine. In the ileum of the small intestine, the digested food is absorbed into the blood and lymph. The digested food then progresses into the large intestine. In the colon, water is reabsorbed. Faeces are then stored in the rectum and leave the alimentary canal via the anus.

Question 25: C

Statement 1 is true.
Statement 2 is true. For example, the drug curare, a South American plant toxin which is used in arrow poison, stops the nerve impulse from crossing the synapse and causes paralysis and can stop breathing.
Statement 3 is false. The sheath provides insulation for the nerve axon and increases the speed of impulse transmission via saltatory conduction.
Statement 4 is false. The peripheral nervous system includes motor and sensory neurons carrying impulses between receptors, effectors, and the central nervous system. The CNS consists of the spinal cord and the brain.
Statement 5 is true. A reflex arc travels from sensory neuron to relay neuron to motor neuron and is an innate mechanism designed to keep the animal safe. For example, it allows a person to quickly draw their hand away from a flame.

Question 26: D

Statement 1 is false because the pulmonary artery carries deoxygenated blood from the right ventricle to the lungs.

Statement 2 is true. This property of the aorta allows it to carry blood at high pressure and is why it pulsates.

Statement 3 is false because the mitral valve, otherwise known as the bicuspid valve, is between the left atrium and left ventricle.

Statement 4 is true.

Question 27: B

Statement 1 is true. Males have one X chromosome so if the allele is present they will be affected. Females have two X chromosomes so both need to be affected to be red-green colour blind as the condition is recessive

Statement 2 is true because according to the Punnett square below half of the children will have the homozygous recessive tt genotype and so will be non-rollers.

	T	t
t	Tt	tt
t	Tt	tt

Statement 3 is true because all of the male children will inherit an X chromosome from the mother which will carry the colour-blind allele.

Question 28: E

Statement 1 is true.

Statement 2 is true. Decomposers in the soil break down urea and the bodies of dead organisms and this results in the production of ammonia in the soil.

Statement 3 is true.

Statement 4 is true.

Question 29: D

Statement 1 is false. Sucrose is a disaccharide formed by the condensation of two monosaccharides (glucose and fructose).

Statement 2 is false. Lactose is a disaccharide formed by condensation of a glucose molecule with a galactose molecule.

Statement 3 is true. Glucose has two isomers: alpha-glucose and beta-glucose.

Statement 4 is true.

Statement 5 is true.

Question 30: F

Alleles are different versions of the same gene. If you are a homozygous for a trait, you have two identical alleles for that particular gene, and if you are heterozygous you have two different alleles of that gene. Recessive traits only appear in the phenotype when there are no dominant alleles for that trait, i.e. two recessive alleles are carried.

Question 31: D

Remember that red blood cells don't have a nucleus and therefore have no DNA. In meiosis, a diploid cell divides in such a way so as to produce four haploid cells. Any type of cell division will require energy.

Question 32: C

The hypothalamus detects too little water in the blood, so the pituary gland releases ADH. The kidney maintains the blood water level, and allows less water to be lost in the urine until the blood water level returns to normal.

Question 33: E

Venous blood has a higher level of carbon dioxide and lower oxygen. Carbon dioxide forms carbonic acid in aqueous solution, thus making the pH of venous blood slightly more acidic than arterial blood. This leaves only E and F as possibilities, but releasing pH levels cannot fluctuate significantly gives pH 7.4.

Question 34: E

The cytoplasm is 80% water, but also contains, among other things, electrolytes and proteins. The cytoplasm doesn't contain everything, e.g. DNA is found in the nucleus.

Question 35: C

ATP is produced in mitochondria in aerobic respiration and in the cytoplasm during anaerobic respiration only.

Question 36: C

The cell membrane allows both active transport and passive transport by diffusion of certain ions and molecules, and is found in eukaryotes and prokaryotes like bacteria. It is a phospholipid bilayer.

Question 37: A

1 and 2 only: 223 PAIRS = 446 chromosomes; meiosis produces 4 daughter cells with half of the original number of chromosomes each, while mitosis produces two daughter cells with the original number of chromosomes each.

Question 38: E

If Bob is homozygous dominant (RR) the probability of having a child with red hair is 0%. However, if Bob is heterozygous (Rr), there is a 50% chance of having a child with red hair, since Mary must be homozygous recessive (rr) to have red hair. As we do not know Bob's genotype, both possibilities must be considered.

Question 39: A

If an offspring is born with red hair, it confirms Bob is heterozygous (Rr). He cannot have a red-haired child if he is homozygous dominant (RR), and would himself have red hair were he homozygous recessive (rr).

Question 40: A

Monohybrid cross rr and Rr results in 50% Rr and 50% rr offspring. 50% of offspring will have black hair, but they will be heterozygous for the hair allele.

Question 41: C

Statement 1 is true.

Statement 2 is false. The transition metals are both malleable and ductile, they conduct heat and electricity and they form positive ions when reacted with non-metals.

Statement 3 is true. Thermal decomposition is a reaction whereby a substance breaks down into two or more other substances due to heat. When a transition metal carbonate is heated, metal oxide and carbon dioxide are produced. The carbon dioxide can be collected and will turn limewater cloudy.

An example of this reaction is: $CuCO_3 \rightarrow CuO + CO_2$

Statement 4 is false. Transition metal hydroxides are insoluble in water.

Statement 5 is true.

Question 42: E

There are 9 Sulphur atoms on the left so there must be 9 on the right. Therefore, the values of B and C must add to make 9. This can be written as an equation: $B+C=9$

It is now useful to try to balance the Oxygen atoms: $4A+36 = 10+4B+4C+14$

Simplify to give: $12 = 4B+4C-4A$

Equation 1 can now be substituted into equation 2 to give: $12 = (4x9)-4A$

$24 = 4A \rightarrow A = 6$

There are 6 Potassium atoms on the left. This means that there must also be 6 potassium atoms on the right, so B must by 3. As shown in equation 1, B and C add to make 9 so C must be 6.

$\underline{5}\ PhCH_3 + \underline{6}\ KMnO_4 + \underline{9}\ H_2SO_4 = \underline{5}\ PhCOOH + \underline{3}\ K_2SO_4 + \underline{6}\ MnSO_4 + \underline{14}\ H_2O$

Question 43: A

This question requires the use of the equation: $C = \frac{n}{v}$ where C= concentration, n= moles and v=volume

Convert $25cm^3$ into litres to get 0.025 litres and plug the values for concentration and volume into the equation to get the number of moles: $0.1 = \frac{n}{0.025}$ so n=0.0025

This question also requires the use of the equation: $n = \frac{m}{Mr}$ where m=mass, n=moles and Mr= molecular mass

The molecular mass is the sum of one calcium and two chlorine atoms which is equal to $111gmol^{-1}$.

Inserting the molecular mass and number of moles into the above equation can be used to calculate the mass of calcium chloride: $m = 0.0025 \ x \ 111 = 0.28g$

Question 44: E

This question requires use of the equation: Percentage yield = $\frac{actual\ yeild\ (g)}{predicted\ yield\ (g)}$ x 100.

If all of the benzene was converted to product (100 percent yield) then 20.5g of nitrobenzene would be produced:

13g C_6H_6 x $\frac{1\ mol\ C6H6}{78g\ C6H6}$ x $\frac{123g\ C6H5NO2}{1\ mol\ C6H5NO2}$ = 20.5g $C_6H_5NO_2$.

However, only 16.4g are actually produced. Using the equation, we can now calculate the percentage yield:

$\frac{16.4g}{20.5g}$ x 100 = 80% yield.

Question 45: E

The question is asking for which of the statements are *false*.

Statement 1 is true.

Statement 2 is true.

Statement 3 is false. Ionic compounds do conduct electricity when dissolved in water or when melted because the ions can move and carry current. On the other hand, solid ionic compounds do not conduct electricity.

Statement 4 is true. Alloys contain different sized atoms, making it harder for the layers of atoms to slide over each other.

Question 46: D

The Ar of Carbon is 12, Hydrogen is 1 and Oxygen is 16. Therefore, 12g of carbon is 1 mole of carbon; 2g of H is 2 moles of hydrogen and 16g of O is 1 mole of oxygen. The empirical formula is therefore CH_2O. The molecular weight is 30 $g.mol^{-1}$, which goes into 120 $g.mol^{-1}$ exactly 4 times. The empirical formula must therefore be multiplied by 4 to obtain the molecular formula so the molecular formula is $C_4H_8O_4$.

Question 47: C

Statement 1 is true.

Statement 2 is false. The melting and boiling points increase as you go down the group.

Statement 3 is true.

Statement 4 is false. Chloride is more reactive than bromine, so no displacement reaction occurs.

Statement 5 is true.

Question 48: F

Ammonia is 1 nitrogen and 3 hydrogen atoms bonded covalently. N = 14g and H = 1g per mole, so percentage of N in NH_3 = 14g/17g = 82%. It can be produced from N_2 through fixation or the industrial Haber process for use in fertiliser, and may break down to its components.

Question 49: A

Milk is weakly acidic, pH 6.5-7.0, and contains fat. This is broken down by lipase to form fatty acids - turning the solution slightly more acidic.

Question 50: C

Glucose loses four hydrogen atoms; one definition of an oxidation reaction is a reaction in which there is loss of hydrogen.

Question 51: C

Isotopes have the same number of protons and electrons, but a different number of neutrons. The number of neutrons has no impact on the rate of reactions.

Question 52: E

$Mg + H_2SO_4 \rightarrow MgSO_4 + H_2$

Number of moles of Mg = $\frac{6}{24}$ = 0.25 moles.

1 mole of Mg reacts with 1 mole H_2SO_4 to produce 1 mole of magnesium sulphate. Therefore, 0.25 moles H_2SO_4 will react to produce 0.25 moles of $MgSO_4$.

M_r of H_2SO_4 = 2 + 32 + 64 = 98g per mole

The mass of H_2SO_4 used = 0.25 moles x 98g per mole = 24.5g.

Since 30g of H_2SO_4 is present, H_2SO_4 is in excess and the magnesium is the limiting reagent.

M_r of $MgSO_4$ = 24 + 32 + 64 = 120g per mole

The mass of $MgSO_4$ produced = 0.25 moles x 120g per mole = 30g which is the same mass as that of sulphuric acid in the original reaction.

Question 53: B

Start by multiplying each term by ax to give: $a(y+x)=x^2+a^2$

Expand the brackets: $ay+ax=x^2+a^2$

Subtract ax from both sides: $ay=x^2+a^2-ax$

Lastly, divide the both sides by a to get: $y = \frac{x^2+a^2-ax}{a}$

Question 54: C

Solve as simultaneous equations. Start by substituting x = $\frac{y}{3}$ into equation B.

This gives y = $\frac{18}{y} - 7$

Multiply every term by y to give:

$0=y^2 +7y - 18$

Factorise this quadratic to give:

$0=(y+9)(y-2)$

Where the graphs meet, y is equal to 2 and 9. Then y=3x so the graphs meet when x = 6 and x = 27

Question 55: B

To win one game, Rupert must win one squash game and one tennis game. In order to calculate the probability one winning one game, it is necessary to add the probability of winning one tennis game and losing one squash game to the probability of losing one tennis game and winning one squash game. The following calculation must be performed: $(\frac{3}{4} \text{ x } \frac{2}{3}) + (\frac{1}{4} \text{ x } \frac{1}{3}) = \frac{7}{12}$

Question 56: C

The numbers can all be written as a fraction over 36:

- $0.\dot{3}$ is the same as $\frac{12}{36}$
- $\frac{11}{18}$ is the same as $\frac{22}{36}$
- 0.25 is the same as $\frac{9}{36}$
- 0.75 is the same as $\frac{27}{36}$
- $\frac{62}{72}$ is the same as $\frac{31}{36}$
- $\frac{7}{7}$ is the same as $\frac{36}{36}$

Ordering them from lowest to highest gives: $\frac{7}{36}$; 0.25; $0.\dot{3}$; $\frac{11}{18}$; 0.75; $\frac{62}{72}$; $\frac{7}{7}$

Therefore, the median value is $\frac{11}{18}$

Question 57: B

This question requires the use of the equation:
p=mv where p=momentum, m=mass and v=velocity.

The total momentum before the collision is equal to the sum of the momentum of carriage 1 (12000 x 5) and carriage 2 (8000 x 0), which is 60,000 kg ms^{-1}. Momentum is conserved before and after the collision so the total momentum after the event also equal 60,000 kg ms^{-1}. The carriages now move together so the combined mass is 20,000kg. Using the equation again, the total momentum (60,000 kg ms^{-1}) divided by the total mass (20,000 kg) gives the velocity of the train carriages after the crash, which is equal to 3 ms^{-1}.

Question 58: C

Statement 1 is true.
Statement 2 is false because infrared has a longer wavelength than visible light.
Statement 3 is true.
Statement 4 is false because gamma radiation and not infrared radiation is used to sterilise food and to kill cancer cells.
Statement 5 is true because darker skins contain a higher amount of melanin pigment, which absorbs UV light.

Question 59: C

Statement 1 is false. In a nuclear reactor, every uranium nuclei split to release energy and three neutrons. An explosion could occur if all the neutrons are absorbed by further uranium nuclei as the reaction would escalate out of control. Control rods that are made of boron absorb some of the neutrons and control the chain reaction.
Statement 2 is false. Nuclear fusion occurs when a deuterium and tritium nucleus are forced together. The nuclei both carry a positive charge and consequently, very high temperatures and pressures are required to overcome the electrostatic repulsion. These temperatures and pressures are expensive and hard to repeat and so fusion is not currently suitable as a source of energy.
Statement 4 is true. During beta decay, a neutron transforms into a proton and an electron. The proton remains in the nucleus, whereas the electron is emitted and is referred to as a beta particle. The carbon-14 nucleus now has one more proton and one less neutron, so the atomic number increases by 1 and the atomic mass number remains the same.
Statement 5 is false. Beta particles are more ionising than gamma rays and less ionising than alpha particles.

Question 60: E

Firstly, deal with the term in the brackets: $3^3=27$

$(x^{½})^3 = x^{1.5}$

$(3x^{½})^3 = 27x^{1.5}$

Next, divide by $3x^2$: $\frac{27}{3} = 9$

$\frac{x^{1.5}}{x^2} = x^{-0.5} = \frac{1}{\sqrt{x}}$

Answer= $\frac{9}{\sqrt{x}}$

END OF PAPER

Mock Paper D Answers

Question 1: B

James runs 26.2 seconds, which is outside the qualifying time, therefore he does not qualify.

Question 2: D

Using s as the sandwich price, c for the crisps and w for the watermelon, the equation to solve is $£5.60 = s + c + w$.

Substituting in the information that $w = 2s$ and $s = 2c$:

$£5.60 = s + 2s + s/2 \quad or\, £5.60 = 3.5\,s$

$s = £1.60$

$Hence, w = 2\,x\,£160 = £320$

Question 3: E

Jane leaves at 2:35pm and arrives at 3:25pm, taking 50 minutes. Sam's journey takes twice as long, so leaving at 3:00pm it takes 100 minutes, giving an arrival time of 4:40pm.

Question 4: C

Find original pay: £250/0.86 = 290 basic original pay. Add the rise: (290 x 1.05) + 6 = £311 new basic pay. Subtract the income tax at 12% = 311 x 0.88 = £273 new pay rate

Question 5: C

Given the first cube is a white cube, you are drawing from one of three boxes, boxes A, C or D. Boxes C and D will have just had their only white cube removed, whereas box A will have one white cube remaining. Therefore the probability of drawing a second white cube is $^1/_3$, thus the probability of non-white (i.e. black) is $^2/_3$.

Question 6: E

This is a simultaneous equations question.

500 + 10(x – 80) = 600 + 5x; true when x ≥ 80.

500 + 10x – 800 = 600 + 5x

» 5x = 900

» x = 180, therefore after 180 minutes

Question 7: E

The keyword here is **efficiency**. Simon's argument is that a slow eater will be less productive. Whilst eating slowly might be a weakness (D) and lunch breaks might be considered a distraction (B), they do not directly support Simon's argument.

Although eating slow may lead to longer lunches (A) and reduce the time available to work (C), this doesn't necessarily mean the individual will be less productive – the lunch break might make them more efficient than other individuals. In order for Simon to assume slow eaters will be less productive, it must follow that slower eaters will have less time to work **efficiently** (E).

Question 8: D

This is a LCM question. We need to find the lowest common multiple of the song lengths. The LCM of 100, 180 and 240 is 3,600 seconds – equal to 60 minutes. For ease of arithmetic, you may choose to work reduce all numbers by a factor of 10.

Question 9: D

The journey is 3 hours and 45 mins, minus a 14 minute break gives 3hrs 31 mins travel time, or 211 minutes. Therefore the average speed is 51mph, or 82kmh by using the stated conversion factor.

Question 10: C
The mean guess is £13.80, which is £5.80 too high.

Question 11: C
The overall error for respondent 3 is £13, which is the least.

Question 12; B
The passage suggests that the attacks were carried out by extra-terrestrial beings. Though the supposed UFO sightings have rational explanations, the writer feels this is insufficient to dismiss his idea.

Question 13: C
The initial argument suggests that two things must be present for an action to happen. If only one is absent, the action cannot happen. Argument C has the same form, the others do not.

Question 14: E
Building model ships requires several positive traits. The passage does not tell us which the most important or most commonly lacked skill is, only that more than one skill is required for success.

Question 15: C
Joseph does not have blue cubic blocks, since all his blue blocks are cylindrical.

Question 16: B
The chance of red is 2/6 = 1/3. To get no reds at all, it must be non-red for each of three independent rolls. The probability of this is $(2/3)^3 = 8/27$. Therefore, the probability of at least one red is 1 – 8/27 = <u>19/27</u>

Question 17: D
These three furniture items are compatible with having 6 legs. All the other statements are false.

Question 18: D
Work this out by time. The friends are closing on each other at a total of 6mph overall, therefore the 42 miles take 7 hours. In seven hours, the falcon, flying at 18mph covers 18 x 7 = 126 miles.

Question 19: C
The passage tells us that antibiotic resistance could lead to people dying from Victorian diseases, and that liberal use of antibiotics in farming is the "most significant" contributor to this. Therefore it would be true to say that this use of antibiotics could cause serious harm.

Question 20: B
Calculate the overall cost of three stationery sets, then subtract any items not bought. For each item shared between two people, there is one of that item not required. The overall cost is £6.00 per person, £18.00 overall. Subtract one geometry set (£3), one paper pad (£1) and one pencil (50p) to give £13.50 overall cost.

Question 21: C
General knowledge question

Question 22: A
General knowledge question

Question 23: E
Haemoglobin is contained within red blood cells and is not free in the blood. Additionally, as a protein it is too large to normally pass through the glomerular filtration barrier. All the other substances are freely filtered.

Question 24: B
In order for the membrane potential to become more positive, there must be a net movement of positive ions into the muscle cell (so it becomes more positive compared to its resting state). Since there is a greater concentration of sodium ions outside, more sodium than potassium must move inwards.

Question 25: F
A polymer consists of repeating monomeric subunits. Polythene consists of multiple ethenes; glycogen of glucose; collagen of amino acids, starch of glucose; DNA of nucleotide bases, but triglycerides are not composed of monomeric subunits.

Question 26: E
Increased ADH causes more water reabsorption. This concentrates the sodium in the urine by reducing urine volume. In the healthy kidney, all glucose is reabsorbed and none is excreted into the urine.

Question 27: D
Diastole is the relaxation phase of the cardiac cycle. In diastole the pressure in the aorta decreases as the contractile force from the ventricles is reduced. All of the other statements are true; the aortic valve closes after ventricular systole. All four chambers of the heart have blood in them throughout the cardiac cycle.

Question 28: B
Competitive inhibition occurs when the inhibitor prevents a reaction by binding to the enzyme active site. Hence, a higher concentration of the substrate can result in the same overall rate of reaction. i.e. the substrate outcompetes the competitor.

Non-competitive inhibition is where the inhibitor binds to the enzyme (not at the active site) and prevents the reaction from taking place. Increasing the substrate concentration therefore does not increase the reaction rate i.e. the substrate cannot outcompete the competitor as the enzymes are disabled and the competitor is not binding to the active site.

In this graph, line 1 shows the normal reaction without inhibition, line 2 shows competitive inhibitor and line 3 shows non-competitive inhibition.

Question 29: E
Nucleic acids are only found in the nucleus (DNA & RNA) and cytoplasm (RNA). They are not a component of the plasma membrane, whereas the other molecules are.

Question 30: D
The main artery to the lungs is the pulmonary artery, which gets blocked. The clot must therefore travel through the inferior vena cava and right side of the heart. It does not enter the superior vena cava or left (systemic) circulation.

Question 31: B
Note that the units are the same ($M = moldm^{-3}$), only the orders of magnitude are different. Convert the orders of magnitude to discover a 10^6 difference with more chloride than thyroxine

Question 32: B
Glycogen is not a hormone, it is a polysaccharide storage product primarily found in muscle and the liver.

Question 33: D
Reflexes can be influenced by the brain e.g. if you willingly pick up a hot plate, you will be able to withstand much greater heat than if you touch it by accident and discover it is hot. Reflex actions are fast as they usually bypass the brain. Since they are mediated by nerves, they are much faster than endocrine responses. Most animals show basic reflexes like the heat-withdrawal reflex which requires both sensory and motor components.

Question 34: D

The key here is to note that the answers are several orders of magnitude apart so you can round the numbers to make your calculations easier:

$Probability\ of\ bacteria\ being\ resistant\ to\ every\ antibiotic\ =$

$P\ (Res\ to\ Antibiotic\ 1) x\ P\ (Res\ to\ Antibiotic\ 2) x\ P\ (Res\ to\ Antibiotic\ 3)\ x\ P\ (Res\ to\ Antibiotic\ 4)$

$= \frac{100}{10^{11}} x \frac{1000}{10^9} x \frac{100}{10^8}\ x \frac{1}{10^5}$

$= \frac{10^8}{10^{33}} = \frac{1}{10^{25}}$

Question 35: A

Producers are found at the bottom of food chains and always have the largest biomass.

Question 36: C

When the chest walls expand, the intra-thoracic pressure decreases. This causes the atmospheric pressure outside the chest to be greater than pressure inside the chest, resulting in a flow of air into the chest.

Question 37: F

All the statements are true; the carbon and nitrogen cycles are examinable in Section 2, so make sure you understand them! The atmosphere is 79% inert N_2 gas, which must be 'fixed' to useable forms by high-energy lightning strikes or by bacterial mediation. Humans also manually fix nitrogen for fertilisers with the Haber process.

Question 38: H

None of the above statements are correct. Mutations can be silent, cause a loss of function, or even a gain in function, depending on the exact location in the gene and the base affected. Mutations only cause a change in protein structure if the amino acids expressed by the gene affected are changed. This is normally due to a shift in reading frame. Whilst cancer arises as a result of a series of mutations, very few mutations actually lead to cancer.

Question 39: C

Remember that heart rate is controlled via the autonomic nervous system, which isn't a part of the central nervous system.

Question 40: H

None of the above are correct. There is no voluntary input to the heart in the form of a neuronal connection. Parasympathetic neurones slow the heart and sympathetic nervous input accelerates heart rate.

Question 41: C

It's important to know your reactivity series as its easy marks. Remember that potassium is more reactive than sodium, as it has a greater number of electron shells, with the outermost single electron being more loosely attracted to the nucleus because of this, and hence more likely to be lost. Following this pattern, sodium is the next most reactive and copper the least.

Question 42: E

144ml of water is 144g, which is the equivalent of 8 moles. 8 times Avogadro's constant gives the number of molecules present, which is $4.8 x 10^{24}$. There are 10 protons and 10 electrons in each water molecule, hence there are $4.8 x 10^{25}$ electrons.

Question 43: F

Write the equation to calculate molar ratios:

$C_8H_{18} + 12.5\ O_2 \rightarrow 8CO_2 + 9H_2O$

Travelling 10 miles uses: 228 x 10 = 2,280g of Octane.

M_r of Octane = 12 x 8 + 18 x 1 = 114

Number of moles of octane used = 2,280/114 = 20 moles. Thus, 160 moles of CO_2 must be produced.

M_r of CO_2 = 12 + 16 x 2= 44

Mass of CO_2 produced = 44 x 160 = 7,040 g = 7.04 kg

Question 44: F

Reactivity series of metals:

Cu is more reactive than Ag and will displace it.

Ca is more reactive than H and will displace it.

2 and 4 are incorrect because Fe is higher in the reactivity series than Cu and Fe is lower in the reactivity series than Ca, so no displacement will occur.

Question 45: G

Moving left to right is the equivalent of moving down the metal reactivity series (i.e. Na is most reactive and Zn is least reactive). Therefore, moving from left to right, the reactivity of the metals decreases, likelihood of corrosion decreases, less energy is required to separate metals from their ores and metals lose electrons less readily to form positive ions.

Question 46: F

Halogens become less reactive as you progress down group 17. Thus in order of increasing reactivity from left to right: I→ Br→ Cl. Therefore, I will not displace Br, Cl will displace Br and Br will displace I.

Question 47: A

Wires are made out of copper because it is a good conductor of electricity. Copper is also used in coins (not aluminium). Aluminium is resistant to corrosion but because of a layer of aluminium oxide (not hydroxide).

Question 48: C

$2Li + 2H_2O \rightarrow 2LiOH + H_2$

Therefore, 2 moles of Li react to produce 1 mole of H_2 gas (24 dm^3).

The number of moles of Li = $\frac{21}{7}$ = 3 moles.

Thus, 1.5 moles of H_2 gas are produced = 36 dm^3.

Question 49: B

$MgCl_2$ contains stronger bonds than NaCl because Mg ions have a 2+ charge, thus having a stronger electrostatic pull for negative chloride ions. The smaller atomic radius also means that the nucleus has less distance between it and incoming electrons. Transition metals are able to form multiple stable ions e.g. Fe^{2+} and Fe^{3+}.

Covalently bonded structures do tend to have lower MPs than ionically bonded, but the giant covalent structures (diamond and graphite for example) have very high melting points. Graphite is an example of a covalently bonded structure which conducts electricity.

Question 50: D

Energy is released from reaction **A**, as shown by a negative enthalpy. The reaction is therefore exothermic. Since energy is released, the product CO_2 has less energy than the reactants did. Therefore, CO_2 is more stable. Reaction **B** has a positive enthalpy, which means energy must be put into the reaction for it to occur i.e. it's an endothermic reaction. That means that the products (CaO and CO_2) have more energy and are less stable than the reactants ($CaCO_3$).

Question 51: B

Solid oxides are unable to conduct electricity because the ions are immobile. Metals are extracted from their molten ores by electrolysis. Fractional distillation is used to separate miscible liquids with similar boiling points. Mg^{2+} ions have a greater positive charge and a smaller ionic radius than Na^+ ions, and therefore have stronger bonds.

Question 52: E

Li^+ (2) and Na^+ (2, 8)

Mg^{2+} (2, 8) and Ne (2, 8)

Na^{2+} (2, 7) and Ne (2, 8)

O^{2-} (2, 4) and a Carbon atom (2, 4)

Question 53: B

Equate the volume with the surface area in the proportion instructed by the question. $3(^4/_3\pi r^3) = 4\pi r^2$, simplifies to r = 1.

Question 54: B

Gravitational potential energy increases as the grain is lifted further from floor; this is equal to the work done against gravity to attain the higher position. The potential energy equal to mgΔh, so it is dependent upon the mass of the grain that is lifted.

Question 55: E

This is a tricky question that requires a conceptual leap. Only the top candidates will get this correct.

Surface Area of Earth $= 4\pi r^2$

$= 4\,x\,\,3\,x\,(0.6\,x\,10^7)^2$

$= 12\,x\,(6\,x\,10^6)^2$

$= 12\,x\,36\,x\,10^{12}$

$= 3.6\,x\,10^{14}$

Since $= \frac{Force}{Area}$, $Atmospheric\ Pressure = \frac{Force\ exerted\ byatmosphere}{Surface\ Area\ of\ Earth}$

Therefore: $Force = 10^5 x\ 3.6\,x\,10^{14} = 3.6\,x\,10^{19}\,N$

The force exerted by the atmosphere is equal to its weight therefore:

$Force = Weight = mass\ x\ g$

Hence, $Atmospheric\ Mass = \frac{3.6\,x\,10^{19}}{10} = 3.6\,x\,10^{18}\,Kg$

Question 56: D

F = ma; therefore the difference in force is equal to $m_1a_1 - m_2a_2$. This equals (6 x 6) – (2 x 8) = 20N

Question 57: B

$Number\ of\ annual\ flights = Flights\ per\ hour\ x\ Number\ of\ hours\ in\ one\ year\ x\ Number\ of\ airports$

$= 4\,x\,(24\,x\,365)\,x\,1000 = 96\,x\,365\,x\,(1000) \approx 100\,x\,365\,x\,10\,x\,100 = 365\,x\,10^5 = 36.5\ Million$

However, this is an overestimate since we have multiplied by 100 instead of 96. Hence, the actual answer will be slightly lower. 35 Million is the only other viable option available.

365x24=8760 is the number of hours in a year, then 8760 x number of flights per hour (4) = 35040 flights per year per airport. Multiply by the number of airports – 42 million to the nearest million.

Question 58: A

Because the two sides of the circuit are in parallel, both sets of lights experience a 24v voltage drop across them. In lights R and S this is shared equally between them, but in lights P and Q, the new light with twice the resistance takes twice the voltage in accordance with Ohm's Law (V= IR).

Question 59: D

Add the first and last equations together to give: 2F = 4, thus F = 2.

Then add the second and third equations to give 2F – 2H= 5. Thus, H = -0.5

Finally, substitute back in to the first equation to give 2 + G – 0.5 = 1. Thus, G = -0.5

Therefore, FGH = 2 x -0.5 x -0.5 = 0.5.

Question 60: E

This is a simple recall question. X rays have the shortest wavelength whilst microwaves have the longest wavelengths with visible light being somewhere in the middle. It is well worth your time remembering the basic positions of the components of the electromagnetic spectrum as it frequently gets tested in the IMAT.

END OF PAPER

Mock Paper E Answers

Question 1: B

The total saving on the final booking relative to the first is £230, but the cost of two cancellations must be deducted (£90) giving a total saving of £140.

Question 2: B

There are originally no odd numbered balls in Bag A. But as a result of the transfer, there could be an odd ball in Bag A. Therefore the probability of drawing an odd ball is found by multiplying the probability of selecting the new ball ($^1/_5$) from Bag A by the probability that that ball is odd ($^2/_5$ – given by adding the one odd ball in the bag C originally to the odd ball introduced from Bag B) giving an probability of $^2/_{25}$ that the selected ball from Bag A is odd.

Question 3: B

Assume the price of bread is 100p. 100 x 1.4 x 0.8 = 112p after the subsidy. The cost of three loaves is therefore 336p (divided four ways this equals 84p per loaf). Hence, as a percentage of the original price, this is 84%.

Question 4: D

At 2120hrs, the minute hand is pointing to 4 and the hour hand is pointing one third of the way past 9 towards 10. 360°/12 = 30° – this is the number of degrees per hour division. Between the two hands then, there are 5 hour divisions plus an extra $^1/_3$. Therefore the angle is (30x5)+(30/3) = 160°

Question 5: B

There is a 3l and 5l bucket – therefore 4 litres can be measured from the difference between the buckets as follows. Fill the 5l bucket, decant 3l into the smaller bucket and then you are left with 2l in the large bucket. Pour this into the tank. Repeat the process again, decanting the remaining 2l into the tank once again to make 4l in total. The first time, 5 litres was required. The second time, the 3 litres from the second bucket could be tipped back into the 5l bucket, and then filled up with fresh water to measure the final 2 litres in. Therefore 4 + 3 = 7 litres of water is sufficient to fill the tank with 4l.

Question 6: D

To answer this question, make a timeline showing the locations of the different genres of books. Place each book on the timeline as appropriate, making sure to indicate where more than one location is a possibility. From that, you will see that literature books are located to the right of engineering. This is true since they are to the right of art (which we know is right of mathematics (and therefore engineering, since the run between the sciences is uninterrupted)). The other statements, whilst potentially true, cannot be deduced for certain.

Question 7: C

The passage tells us that brand new cars lose value quickly, despite the car being virtually unchanged. Therefore in the absence of any contradictory information, it is reasonable to conclude that buying second hand cars is a wise choice.

Question 8: B

First, calculate how many bottles are sold. 2000 – (2000x0.9x0.8) = 560 bottles. Then divide the total profit by the number of units to give the profit per unit, which comes to 11200/560 = £20 per bottle.

Question 9: E

The definition of timelessness requires something to be tested by time. Something that modern furniture cannot fulfil. Therefore statement E expresses a significant flaw in the reasoning. The other statements do not refer to the 'timelessness' aspect of furniture, therefore they are not directly relevant to the argument.

Question 10: A

The passage talks about the benefits of drinking red wine, not about living near to vineyards. The passage does not state that Italians drink more wine than Germans, therefore the assumption that they do is central to the argument.

Question 11: C

Tom arrives at 1620, and leaves 45 mins after Jane leaves. Therefore he also leaves 45 mins after Hannah leaves, since Jane and Hannah leave together. Since his journey is 10 mins faster than Hannah's, he arrives only 35 minutes after Hannah arrives (which happens to be 1620). Therefore Hannah arrives 35 minutes earlier than this, at 1545. Since she left at 1430, her journey took 75 minutes. Jane's journey took 40% longer (1.4 x 75 = 105 minutes). Therefore leaving at the same time as Hannah, 1430, Jane arrived 105 minutes later at 1615.

Question 12: B

This is a simultaneous equations question. Let **x** be the number of standard tickets sold, and **y** be the number of premium tickets sold.

Therefore: $x + y = 600$; $10x + 16y = 6{,}600$

$x = 600 - y$ » substitute: $10(600 - y) + 16y = 6600$

$6y = 600$

$y = 100$, therefore 100 premium tickets were sold.

Question 13: C

Between 20th January and 23rd May, there are 123 days. In 123 days, the moon makes 123/28 = 4.39 orbits. This is equal to 4.39 x 360° = 1580°

Question 14: E

You are looking for a strong opposition to the proposition that students at drama academies are not taught well academically. The strongest opposition would be evidence that such students perform academically well in some objective measure. Evidence of significantly above average GCSE results provides this.

Question 15: D

You should definitely draw this one out on paper. Trace out the paths and you find that both people have a net displacement of 11km to the North. Therefore since Anil is only net 2km East, and Suresh is 17km East of the starting point, there is a 15km separation between them

Question 16: A

Walking at 4mph, 3 miles takes ¾ hour = 45 mins. Adding the 5 minute stop, Chris will arrive at 1820, since he set off at 1730. At 24mph, 6 miles takes ¼ hour, 15 mins. Therefore setting off at 1810, Sarah will arrive at Laura's at 1825. Therefore Chris arrives 5 minutes earlier than Sarah.

Question 17: D

The passage tells us that illegal downloads are causing harm to the music industry. Whilst it gives an example, this does not mean the stated example is the principal issue. The conclusion that best fits the passage as a whole is to say illegal downloading is more harmful than many people think, given their willingness to undertake it.

Question 18: E

First, calculate the amount of water needed for each type of fire. Use algebra:

Use x as the amount of water used to extinguish a house fire. 40,000L = 2x , so x = 20,000L. Then, take y as the amount of water needed to extinguish a garden fire, so 70,000L = 2x + 3y. 30,000L = 3y, y= 10,000L.

Knowing this, A is correct, B is correct, C is correct and D is correct. Only E is false.

Three house and ten garden fires require 160,000 litres to extinguish, not 140,000.

Question 19: D

The passage only talks about people's opinions on the scheme, and not about any action which could potentially be taken. Therefore the best summary is to say that more people oppose the scheme than support it.

Question 20: B + E

The question asks for two responses, therefore you must mark two and get them both correct for one mark. The suggestion is made that reducing wild fishing will improve fish populations. This assertion carries two major assumptions – that the fishing originally caused the decline, and that the decline is reversible, and can therefore recover if the threat is removed. Select these two responses for a mark.

Question 21: D

General knowledge question

Question 22: E

General knowledge question

Question 23: F

None of the above, they are all true facts about digestion.

Question 24: D

Blood flow to the kidneys is constant - not exercise dependent. Overall cardiac output increases since heart rate and stroke volume increase (because there is greater oxygen demand from exercising muscle). There is more blood flow to the muscles to fuel them and to the skin to help lose excess heat. Blood flow to the gut decreases to increase availability to muscles. Blood flow to vital organs such as the kidney and brain remains constant.

Question 25: A

Since A-T and C-G are the DNA base pairings, 29.6% Adenine implies 29.6% Thymine as well. Therefore the remaining 100 – 59.2 = 40.8% is shared between Guanine and Cytosine equally, so there is <u>20.4%</u> cytosine.

Question 26: C

Since CO binds to the oxygen binding site of haemoglobin, it reduces oxygen binding and therefore oxygen carrying capacity of blood. Hence, the blood becomes less oxygenated. Since more blood needs to flow to deliver the same amount of oxygen, this must be accomplished by an increased in heart rate. Haemoglobin does not become heavier as the CO binds **instead** of oxygen rather than in **addition** to. Carbon Dioxide is carried in plasma so is unaffected by carbon monoxide poisoning which affects haemoglobin.

Question 27: E

The most effective method in minimising side effects would be to only target bacteria. Only bacteria have a flagellum.

Question 28: F

Structure A is the right semi-lunar valve, the pulmonary valve. It opens in systole to allow flow of blood from the right ventricle into the pulmonary artery and to the lungs. It closes in diastole to ensure the right ventricle fills only from the right atrium, maintaining a one-way flow of blood. Therefore F is true, it opens when the right atrium is emptying. None of the other statements are true.

Question 29: E

E is the correct sequence. Remember sensory neurone take sensory information to the brain, and motor neurones take information away.

Question 30: B

Intra-thoracic volume must decrease during expiration. Thus, the intercostal muscles relax causing the ribs must move down and in. The diaphragm moves up as well.

Question 31: B

If lipase is not working, fat from the diet will not be broken down, and will build up in the stool. Lactase, for instance, is responsible for breaking down lactose, and its malfunctioning causes lactose-intolerance.

Question 32: F

Oxygenated blood flows from the lungs to the heart via the pulmonary vein. The pulmonary artery carries deoxygenated blood from the heart to the lungs. Animals like fish have single circulatory systems. Deoxygenated blood is found in the superior vena cava, returning to the heart from the body. Veins in the arms and hands frequently don't have valves.

Question 33: E

Enzymatic digestion takes place throughout the GI tract, including in the mouth (e.g. amylase), stomach (e.g. pepsin), and small intestine (e.g. trypsin). The large intestine is primarily responsible for water absorption, whilst the rectum acts as a temporary store for faecal matter (i.e. digestion has finished by the rectum).

Question 34: B

This is an example of the monosynaptic stretch reflex; these reflexes are performed at the spinal level and therefore don't involve the brain.

Question 35: A

Statement 2 describes diffusion, as CO_2 is moving with the concentration gradient. Statement 3 describes active transport, as amino acids are moving against the concentration gradient.

Question 36: I

3 is the correct equation for animals, and 4 is correct for plants.

Question 37: C

The mitochondria are only the site for aerobic respiration, as anaerobic respiration occurs in the cytoplasm. Aerobic respiration produces more ATP per substrate than anaerobic respiration, and therefore is also more efficient. The chemical equation for glucose being respired aerobically is: $C_6H_{12}O_6 + 6O_2 \rightarrow 6CO_2 + 6H_2O$. Thus, the molar ratio is 1:6 (i.e. each mole glucose produces 6 moles of CO_2).

Question 38: B

The nucleus contains the DNA and chromosomes of the cell. The cytoplasm contains enzymes, salts and amino acids in addition to water. The plasma membrane is a bilayer. Lastly, the cell wall is indeed responsible for protecting vs. increased osmotic pressures.

Question 39: D

When a medium is hypertonic relative to the cell cytoplasm, it is more concentrated than the cytoplasm, and when it is hypotonic, it is less concentrated. So, when a medium is hypotonic relative to the cell cytoplasm, the cell will gain water through osmosis. When the medium is isotonic, there will be no net movement of water across the cell membrane. Lastly, when the medium is hypertonic relative to the cell cytoplasm, the cell will lose water by osmosis.

Question 40: A

Stem cells have the ability to differentiate and produce other kinds of cells. However, they also have the ability to generate cells of their own kind and stem cells are able to maintain their undifferentiated state. The two types of stem cells are embryonic stem cells and adult stem cells. The adult stem cells are present in both children and adults.

Question 41: E

Recall that reduction is the gain of electrons whilst oxidation is a loss. Also remember that oxidation the gain of oxygen, while reduction is loss. Only Iodine is gaining electrons and so shows reduction.

Question 42: F

To balance the equation, start working from what you're given – the oxygen. Since you know there are 15 oxygen atoms on the right, there must be the same on the left. Therefore **w** = 5. You also know that there are 30 Hydrogen atoms on the right hand side, and so you can work out x. 30-5 leaves 25 atoms unaccounted for, so x=25.

Question 43: F

The information given can only be used to work out the empirical formula. You would need to know the molar mass in order to calculate the chemical formula.

Question 44: B

The trick in this question is to conserve your units to prevent silly mistakes from creeping in. $200\ cm^{-3} = 0.2\ dm^{-3}$

$Number\ of\ moles = concentration\ x\ volume$ so: $0.2\ x\ 1.8 = 0.36\ mol$

Question 45: E

Group 6 elements are non-metals whilst group 3 elements are metals. Thus, the group 3 element must lose electrons when it reacts with the group 6 element. The donation of electrons from its outer shell will decrease atomic size.

Question 46: B

Reactivity of both group 1 and 2 increases as you go down the groups because the valence electrons that react are further away from the positively charged nucleus (which means the electrostatic attraction between them is weaker). Group 1 metals are usually more reactive because they only need to donate one electron, whilst group 2 metals must donate two electrons.

Question 47: D

This is a straightforward question that tests basic understanding of kinetics. Catalysts help overcome energy barriers by reducing the activation energy necessary for a reaction.

Question 48: D

H^1 contains 1 proton and no neutrons. Isotopes have the same numbers of protons, but different numbers of neutrons. Thus, H^3 contains two more neutrons than H^1.

Question 49: D

These statements all come from the Kinetic Theory of Gases, an idealised model of gases that allows for the derivation of the ideal gas law. The angle at which gas molecules move is not related to temperature; movement is random. Gas molecules lose no energy when they collide with each other, collisions are assumed elastic. The average kinetic energy of gas molecules is the same for all gases at the same temperature as they are assumed to be point masses. Momentum = mass x velocity. Therefore, the momentum of gas molecules increases with pressure as a greater force is exerted on each molecule.

Question 50: D

Oxidation is the loss of electrons and reduction is the gain of electrons (therefore increasing electron density). Halogens tend to act as electron recipients in reactions and are therefore good oxidising agents.

Question 51: E

An exothermic reaction is defined as a chemical reaction that releases energy. Thus, aerobic respiration producing life energy, the burning of magnesium, and the reacting of acids/bases are almost always exothermic processes. Similarly, the combustion of most things (including hydrogen) is exothermic. Evaporation of water is a physical process in which no chemical reaction is taking place.

Question 52: E

$2\ C_3H_6 + 9\ O_2 \rightarrow 6\ H_2O + 6\ CO_2$

Assign the oxidation numbers for each element:

For C_3H_6: C = -2; H = +1

For O_2: O = 0

For H_2O: H = +1; O = -2

For CO_2: C = +4; O = -2

Look for the changes in the oxidation numbers:

H remained at +1

C changed from -2 to +4. Thus, it was oxidized

O changed from 0 to -2. Thus, it was reduced.

Question 53: D

Firstly, convert Litres → m^3: 950 Litres = 0.95 m^3

Buoyancy Force = Volume x Density x g.

= 0.95 x 1000 x 10 = 9,500 N

Weight of the boat = mg= 600 x 10 = 6,000 N

Since buoyancy force > Weight, the boat will float.

The difference between Buoyancy Force + weight = 9500 – 6000 = 3,500N

Hence adding mass of 350kg (=3,500N as *g* is 10) will balance both forces.

Adding further mass will cause the boat to sink. Hence, the answer is 355kg (350kg won't cause sinking – merely balance the force).

Question 54: A

Remember that you can separate the vertical and horizontal components of both bullets. Both bullets actually have zero vertical velocity at t=0. Thus, only gravity affects them- and it does so equally. Therefore, rather counter-intuitively, they hit the floor at the same time.

Question 55: C

You don't need to know the mass of the fish for this one, since there is no acceleration or deceleration taking place. The resistive forces are equivalent to the force of thrust of the fish. Recall that work done = force x distance. Travelling at $2ms^{-1}$, the fish travels 60 seconds x 60 minutes x 2 ms^{-1} = 7200 m in one hour. Therefore the work done against resistive forces is f x d = 2N x 7200 = <u>14,400J</u>

Question 56: D

A Moment of force = Force x Perpendicular distance to pivot

If the lifting arm is a uniform 5m long, the weight exerts $2000\ x\ 10\ x\ 5\ =\ 100{,}000\ Nm$ of torque. In addition, there is a $250\ x\ 10\ x\ 2.5\ =\ 6{,}250\ Nm$ contribution from the weight of the beam ($\frac{5}{7}$ the mass, acting through the centre of mass of the beam).

On the other side, the remaining $\frac{2}{7}$ of the beam makes a $100\ x\ 10\ x\ 1\ =\ 1{,}000\ Nm$ contribution.

Therefore, the counterbalance must make a $(100{,}000\ +\ 6{,}250) - 1{,}000\ =\ 105{,}250\ Nm$ contribution. As the counterbalance arm is 2 m long, this requires a weight of $\frac{105{,}250}{2}\ =\ 52{,}625\ N$ weight, or a mass of 5,263 kg.

The crane's height is a distracter and not needed for this question

Question 57: B

Work out the total energy transferred - 20 x 50W =1,000W of overall power by the 20 strings of lights when on. As W = Js^{-1}, can use the time the lights are on to find the energy used over this time period. 8pm – 6am is 10 hours, so in seconds is 10x60x60 = 36,000s. When multiplying this by the power of all sets of lights, gives the energy used as:

1000 W x 36,000 s = 36,000,000 J of energy, or 36,000kJ. Multiply this by 20 to account for the lights being on for 20 days = gives 720,000 kJ

As 100 kJ of energy costs 2p, need to do 720,000/100 = 7,200. Multiply this by 2p = 14,400p. Convert to pounds by dividing by 100 = **£144.**

Question 58: C

The formula for the sum of internal angles in a regular polygon is given by: $180(n-2)$, where n is the number of sides of the polygon.

Thus: $180(n-2)\ =\ 150\ x\ n$

$180n - 360\ =\ 150n$

$3n\ =\ 36$

$n =\ 12$

Each side is 15cm so the perimeter is 12 x 15cm = 180cm.

Question 59: E

For Resistors in parallel, $\frac{1}{R_T} = \frac{R_1 \, x \, R_2 ...}{R_1 + R_2 ...}$

For the first segment: $\frac{1}{R} = \frac{1}{Z} + \frac{1}{Z} = \frac{2}{Z}$

For the second segment: $\frac{1}{R} = \frac{1}{Z} + \frac{1}{Z} + \frac{1}{Z} = \frac{3}{Z}$

For the third segment: R = Z

Thus the total resistance is: $Z + \frac{Z}{2} + \frac{Z}{3} = 22.$

$\frac{6Z + 3Z + 2Z}{6} = 22$

$11Z = 22 \, x \, 6$

$Z = \frac{132}{11} = 12M\Omega$

Question 60: B

The volume of candle burned in 0.5 hour = $0.5 \, x \, (\pi \, x \, 2^2) = 6cm^{-3}$

$6cm^{-3} = 6 \, x \, 10^{-3} \, m^3$

Since $Density = \frac{mass}{volume}$, in this case 900 $kgm^{-3} = \frac{mass}{6 \, x \, 10^{-3} \, m^3}$

Thus, Mass burned = $900 \, x \, 6 \, x \, 10^{-3} = 5400 \, x \, 10^{-3} kg = 5.4 \, g$

The Mr of $C_{24}H_{52}$ = $12 \, x \, 24 + 52 \, x \, 1 = 340.$

Thus the number of moles burned = $\frac{5.4}{340} = 0.016 \, moles.$

Total Energy transferred = $0.016 \, x \, 11{,}000$

$= 16 \, x \, 10^{-3} \, x \, 11 \, x \, 10^3 = 11 \, x \, 16$

$= 176 \, kJ = 175{,}000 \, J$

END OF PAPER

Mock Paper F Answers

Question 1: D

C is completely irrelevant, so is not a flaw. B is not a flaw because when assessing an argument, anything that is stated (i.e. not concluded from other reasons in the passage) is accepted as true. We do not require evidence or sources for any statistics presented. A and E are both claiming that something is immoral, which is thus expressing an opinion on the part of the arguer. This is not a flaw, the arguer is at liberty to claim something is immoral, and to claim that the government is morally obliged to act, and that it has not done so. Also, E claims that *arguably* this is the most outrageous flaw of the government, clearly expressing an opinion, which is thus not required to be supported. However, D identifies a valid flaw. The argument rests on us accepting that if there were less uninsured drivers, there would be less crashes. This is not necessarily correct, so D is a flaw in the passage.

Question 2: A

The sentence 'Thus, the situation in Brazil is not applicable to the UK, and legalising gun ownership in the UK would be a bad move' gives the main conclusion of the argument and this is summarised in A.B is partially supported by the passage, but the main conclusion concerns the situation in the UK and the passage states that there is little black market in the UK. C is incorrect as the passage only talks about gun ownership, not violent crime more generally. D is not fully supported by the passage, which states only that legalising guns would result in it being *easier* for criminals to acquire guns, not that there would be a large increase in their number. E is not the main conclusion as it focuses on an aspect of the evidence from Brazil, rather than the main conclusion which focuses on gun legislation in the UK.

Question 3: C

For each of the walls where there is no door, the wall is 6 tiles high and 5 tiles wide, which is 30 tiles. The wall where the door is requires a row of 2 tiles above the door, then there is a width of wall of 120cm which requires completely tiling, which is 6 tiles high and 3 tiles wide, hence this wall requires a total of 20 tiles. Hence a total of 110 tiles are required for the walls. The floor is 2 metres by 2 metres, so 5 tiles by 5 tiles, hence 25 tiles are required for the floor. Hence the answer is 135.

Question 4: D

E is irrelevant to which of Trevor and Jane will arrive first, so does not weaken the conclusion. A, B and C all strengthen the answer, giving further reasons why we might expect Trevor to arrive first. D, however, would slow Trevor down, meaning that it was more likely that Jane would arrive first. Thus, D weakens the passage's conclusion, and hence D is the answer.

Question 5: B

Let the number of minutes the journey takes be t. Therefore, ABC charge 400+15t pence for the journey. We can calculate that XYZ taxis charge 400+(30x6) pence, = 580 pence. Therefore, for both journeys to cost the same, 580=400+15t. 180=15t, therefore t=12. Therefore the 6 mile journey needs to take 12 minutes. 6 miles in 12 minutes is 30 miles per hour, so the answer is B.

Question 6: E

We can see that all of answers A through D are essential for the conclusion to be valid from the squire's reasoning. Lancelot must have great courage, this must be a requirement for the Adzol, and no other knights must have sufficient courage, in order for us to be certain that Lancelot will succeed but all of Arthur's other knights will fail. Thus, A and B can be clearly identified as assumptions. C and D require a bit more thought, but we can see that nothing in the passage explicitly states the Elders' tales are correct. If the elders are not correct, then great courage may not be required to be successful in the Adzol. Thus, both C and D are also assumptions. Hence, the answer is E.

Question 7: A

He can prepare each batch of cakes while the previous one is in the oven but it takes longer so we have to allow 25 minutes for each batch, plus 20 minutes for the last batch to cook while no further batch is being prepared. There are 12 in each batch, so for 100 cupcakes there needs to be 9 batches. Hence the total time needed is 25 minutes x 9, + 20 minutes. This is 245 minutes, or 4 hours 5 minutes. Hence to be ready by 4pm he needs to start at 11:55am, so the answer is A.

Question 8: E

B is incorrect, as the passage does not say that arch-shaped gaps *always* indicate where windows once stood, simply that *these arches* do. C is also incorrect, as the passage simply states that windows are not found in *underground halls*. A is a reason in the passage and is not a conclusion. D and E could both be described as conclusions from this passage, but we see that if we accept D as true (along with the fact that the hall is now underground), we have good reason to believe that E is true, whereas E being true does not necessarily mean that D is true. Thus, E is the *main* conclusion, whilst D is an *intermediate conclusion*, which supports the main conclusion.

Question 9: B

E is an irrelevant statement that says nothing about whether England *do* have good players. Answers A and D actually weaken the sporting director's arguments, suggesting that England may have a good team, and it may just be poor performances in world cups, and not a lack of talented players. This leaves B and C. C may appear to strengthen the sporting director's argument, but on closer inspection we see that in fact it says that for the last 70 years, England have had at least 1 player in the top 10 in the world. This does *not* strengthen the argument that England have been lacking talent for the last 25 years, and may actually reinforce the chairman's argument that it is simply the *current* crop of players that are not good enough. Answer B, however, does strengthen the argument, suggesting that England's performances have been poor over the last 20 years, thus strengthening the argument that there may be a lack of talented players that has been ongoing for a couple of decades, as claimed by the sporting director.

Question 10: D

Usually bread rolls cost 30p for a pack, but if the cost per bread roll is reduced by 1p then they will cost 24p. Hence we need to find z, where 24(z+1)=30z, where z is the original number of packs that could have been afforded. 24z+24=30z, hence 24=6z, so z=4. Hence he was originally supposed to be buying 4 packets of bread rolls, which is 6 x 4 = 24 rolls.

Question 11: D

We can first work out the rate of girls' absenteeism. First we need to work out how many of the pupils at Heather Park Academy and Holland Wood Comprehensive are girls. Let g be the number of girls in Heather Park Academy. Then 0.06(g)+0.05(1000-g)=(1000)(0.056). Then 0.06g-0.05g=56-50. Then 0.01g=6, so g = 600. Hence 600 pupils at Heather Park Academy are girls. The proportions at Holland Wood Comprehensive are the same but there are half as many pupils, so 900 pupils at the two schools combined are girls.

The average absenteeism of girls is 7%. We know that 900 of the 1100 girls have an average absenteeism rate of 6%. Let the average absenteeism rate of girls at Hurlington Academy be r. Then 900 x 0.06 +200r = 0.07x1100. Hence 54+200r=77. 77-54 = 200r. 23/200 = r. r=0.115. Hence, the rate of absenteeism amongst girls at Hurlington Academy is 11.5%

Question 12: B

A and E are not relevant, because neither affect the strength of the councillor's argument from a critical thinking point of view. The councillor's argument says nothing about house prices, simply the cost of building the estate and the effects on wildlife, so A is not relevant. E is not relevant because additional support, or likelihood that it will be heeded, does nothing to affect the strength of a given argument. C and D actually strengthen the councillor's argument, suggesting that brownfield land does have good infrastructure (C) and that the greenbelt areas do have a lot of wildlife (D). B does weaken the councillor's argument, as it suggests that building on brownfield land may also have adverse impacts on wildlife.

Question 13: A

B is not a valid conclusion from the passage, because the fact that someone uses an illogical argument (as some pescatarians are claimed to in this passage) does not mean that they cannot use logic. D and E are not conclusions from this passage because the passage is not saying anything about the ethicality of eating meat, but simply commenting that one argument used against doing so is not logical. C and A are both valid conclusions from the passage, but we see that if we accept C as being true, it gives us good cause to believe that A is true, but this does not apply the other way round. Thus, C is an intermediation conclusion, whilst A is the main conclusion.

Question 14: E

The research conducted does not ask about whether it is *important* to learn some of the language before travelling abroad, simply whether participants *would*, so B cannot be concluded. D is incorrect because the passage states *15%* would, which is clearly not less than 10%. The passage states that this is symptomatic of a deeper underlying issue, but does not say that many issues of racism stem from this, so C cannot be concluded. Now, the passage states that 60% of people feel foreign people should learn English before travelling to Britain, and 15% of people would attempt to learn the language before travelling to a country which did not speak English. However, this 15% could be some of the same people as the 60%, in which case A would be incorrect. Thus, A cannot be reliably concluded. However, there must be at least 45% of people who feel that foreign people should learn English, but would not learn a foreign language themselves, so E *can* be reliably concluded.

Question 15: D

She needs to print 400 x 2 = 800 double sided A4 sheets, which will cost 0.01 x 2 x 1.5 = £0.03 each. Hence the total cost of this is 800 x 0.03 = £24. She also needs to print 1500 single sided A5 sheets, costing £0.01 each, giving a total of 1500 x 0.01 = £15. Hence the total cost is £39.

Question 16: B

The passage has stated that if Kirkleatham win the game they will win the league, so E is not an assumption. Meanwhile, the manager has stated A, C and D, and the passage has not claimed anything about whether Kirkleatham can easily win the game, so A and D are not assumptions. However, B does identify an assumption in the passage. The fact that Kirkleatham will not win the game without playing with desire and commitment does *not* mean that they will win the game if they do play with desire and commitment. And we can see that for the argument's conclusion (that Kirkleatham *will* definitely win the league) to be valid from its reasoning, this is required to be true. Thus, B identifies an assumption in the passage.

Question 17: C

A, B, D and E are all directly stated in the passage, so can all be reliably concluded. Perhaps the trickiest of these to see is answer D, which is true because the passage says "*due to*" the advent of more accurate technology, thus clearly identifying that this had *caused* the switch to the situation of most watches being made by machine. C, however, is *not* necessarily true. The passage states that most *watches* are produced by machines, but only states that *some* watchmakers now only perform repairs. This does not necessarily mean that most watchmakers do not produce watches. It could be that only a handful are required in the entirety of the watch industry for repairs, and that the numbers still producing watches exceeds those in the repair business. Thus, C cannot be reliably concluded from the passage.

Question 18: B

A large pizza wish mushrooms and ham is £12, garlic bread is £3, chips are £1.50 x 2 = £3, a dip is £1, hence the current total is £19. The cheapest way to order this is to get the price up to exactly £30 as this will reduce the price to £18. This takes £11. Only one of these options costs £11, which is a large pizza with mushroom. Hence the answer is B.

Question 19: B

We can tell the amounts for the green party and the blue party are both 1/3 of the total, and that the amount for the red party is 1/4 of the total. Hence 1/12 is left, so the amount for the yellow party must be 1/12. Hence the red party have 3 times the intended vote of the yellow party.

Question 20: E

In Rovers' first 3 games, they have scored 1 goal and had 8 goals scored against them. In total they scored 1 goal and had 10 goals scored against them, so they must have lost their last game against United 2-0. In City's first 3 games, they scored 7 goals and had 3 goals scored against them. In total they scored 10 goals and had 4 goals scored against them, so they must have won their game against United 3-1. Hence the answer is E.

Question 21: E

General knowledge question

Question 22: A

General knowledge question

Question 23: G

The replacement of dying, damaged, and lost cells, the growth of the embryonic cell to a multi-cellular organism, and asexual reproduction are the three main reasons why cells divide through mitosis.

Question 24: E

Blood pressure in the aorta is the highest of any vessel in the body, as blood has just been ejected from the left ventricle to go to the body. The pressure in the left ventricle (and hence the Aorta) is higher than that in the right ventricle (and hence the Pulmonary Artery) because the pressure must be sufficient to pump to the entire body, rather than just the lungs.

Question 25: C

A sensory receptor (1) senses the heat of the pan. This information is passed down the sensory neurone (2) through a relay neurone to the motor neurone (4), which then causes the muscle (5) to contract, pulling the finger away.

Question 26: C

The receptor is directly coupled to the sensory neurone, so the communication here is electrical. All information between neurones passes via synapses, which use neurotransmitters to convey the information chemically. This occurs between the sensory neurone and the relay neurone, and between the relay neurone and the motor neurone. Therefore, the answer is C).

Question 27: C

Increasing the concentration of the reactants (not products) would affect reaction rate, which can be monitored by measuring the gas volume released (proportional to molar concentration). This is the reaction for photosynthesis, which does not occur spontaneously and is endothermic.

Question 28: D

Taking the diseased allele to be X^D and X as the normal allele, we can model the scenario in the Punnett square below:

		Carrier Mother	
		X^D	X
Diseased Father	X^D	X^DX^D	X^DX
	Y	X^DY	XY

Boys are XY and girls are XX. 50% of the boys produced would have DMD. So the probability that both boys would have the disease is 0.5 x 0.5 = 0.25

Question 29: E

We can see from the Punnett square that the probability of having a girl with DMD is 25% (X^DX^D). The probability that both are girls with DMD is 0.25 x 0.25 = 0.125.

Question 30: B

All of the following statements are examples of natural selection, except for the breeding of horses. Breeding and animal husbandry are notable methods of artificial selection, which are brought about by humans.

Question 31: C

Chemical reactions take place in the cytoplasm, and the mitochondrion is the site for aerobic respiration releasing energy. The lack of a cell wall means that this is an animal cell.

Question 32: D

White blood cells can engulf/phagocytose pathogens in order to kill them. CO_2 is transported in the plasma, not in blood cells.

Question 33: C

Enzymes create a stable environment to stabilise the transition state. Enzymes do not distort substrates. Enzymes generally have little effect on temperature directly. Lastly, they are able to provide alternative pathways for reactions to occur.

Question 34: C

A negative feedback system seeks to minimise changes in a system by modulating the response in accordance with the error that's generated. Salivating before a meal is an example of a feed-forward system (i.e. salivating is an anticipatory response). Throwing a dart does not involve any feedback (during the action). pH and blood pressure are both important homeostatic variables that are controlled via powerful negative feedback mechanisms, e.g. massive haemorrhage leads to compensatory tachycardia.

Question 35: A

One of the major functions of white blood cells is to defend the body against bacterial and fungal infections. They can kill pathogens by engulfing them and also use antibodies to help them recognise pathogens. Antibodies are produced by white blood cells.

Question 36: B

The CV system does indeed transport nutrients and hormones. It also increases blood flow to exercising muscles (via differential vasodilatation) and also helps with thermoregulation (e.g. vasoconstriction in response to cold). The respiratory system is responsible for oxygenating blood.

Question 37: C

Adrenaline always increases heart rate and is almost always released during sympathetic responses. It travels primarily in the blood and affects multiple organ systems. It is also a potent vasoconstrictor.

Question 38: B

Protein synthesis occurs in the cytoplasm. Proteins are usually coded by several amino acids. Red blood cells lack a nucleus and, therefore, the DNA to create new proteins. Protein synthesis is a key part of mitosis, as it allows the parent cell to grow prior to division.

Question 39: F

Remember that most enzymes work better in neutral environments (amylase works even better at slightly alkaline pH). Thus, adding sodium bicarbonate will increase the pH and hence increase the rate of activity. Adding carbohydrate will have no effect, as the enzyme is already saturated. Adding amylase will increase the amount of carbohydrate that can be converted per unit time. Increasing the temperature to 100° C will denature the enzyme and reduce the rate.

Question 40: E

Taking the normal allele to be C and the diseased allele to be c, one can model the scenario with the following Punnett square:

		Carrier Mother	
		C	**c**
Diseased Father	**c**	Cc	cc
	c	Cc	cc

The gender of the children is irrelevant as the inheritance is autosomal recessive, but we see that all children produced would inherit at least one diseased allele.

Question 41: A

This is an example of an addition reaction: the chloride and hydrogen atoms are added at the unsaturated bond of the but-2-ene, which is between the 2nd and the 3rd C-atom. If you're unsure about this type of question draw it out and the answer will be obvious.

Question 42: C

The electrolysis reaction for brine is: $2\,NaCl + 2\,H_2O = 2\,NaOH + H_2 + Cl_2$

Thus, keeping in mind the stoichiometry of the given equation, the solution must be C.

Question 43: A

If the two isotopes were in equal abundance, the A_r would be 77, half-way between the two isotope masses (the average). The A_r is 76.5 (a weighted average), one quarter of the way between the isotopes, so there must be three times as much of the lighter isotope to move the A_r closer to its mass of 76 (0.75x76 + 0.25x78 = 76.5).

Though there is more of ^{76}X than ^{78}X, this does not necessarily imply that ^{78}X is lost through decay, as opposed to naturally less abundant from the beginning, so there is no way to know the relative stability of the isotopes.

Question 44: C

Increasing the concentration of the reactants (not products) would affect reaction rate, which can be monitored by measuring the gas volume released (proportional to molar concentration). This is the reaction for photosynthesis, which does not occur spontaneously and is endothermic.

Question 45: H

Most polymers are made up of alkenes, which are unsaturated molecules. Polymerisation does not release water, as it is an addition reaction. Depending on the monomer molecule, polymers can take a variety of shapes.

Question 46: B

The equation for the reaction is: $Zn + CuSO_4 \rightarrow ZnSO_4 + Cu$

Assign oxidation numbers for each element:

For Zn: Zn = 0

For $CuSO_4$: Cu = +2; S = +6; O = -2

For $ZnSO_4$: Zn = +2; S = +6; O = -2

For Cu: Cu = 0

With these oxidation numbers, we can see that Zn was oxidized and Cu in $CuSO_4$ was reduced. Thus, Zn acted as the reducing agent and Cu in $CuSO_4$ is the oxidizing agent.

Question 47: B

Acids are proton donors which only exist in aqueous solution, which is a liquid state. Strong acids are fully ionised in solution and the reaction between an acid and a base → salt + water.

The pH of weak acids is usually between 4 and 6.

Question 48: G

Let x be the relative abundance of Z^6 and y the relative abundance of Z^8.
The average atomic mass takes the abundances of all 3 isotopes into account.
Thus, (Abundance of Z^5)(Mass Z^5) + (Abundance of Z^6)(Mass Z^6) + (Abundance of Z^8)(Mass Z^8) = 7
Therefore: $(5 \times 0.2) + 6x + 8y = 7$
So: $6x + 8y = 6$
Divide by two to give: $3x + 4y = 3$
The abundances of all isotopes = 100% = 1
This gives: $0.2 + x + y = 1$
Solve the two equations simultaneously:
$y = 0.8 - x$
$3x + 4(0.8 - x) = 3$
$3x + 3.2 - 4x = 3$
Therefore, $x = 0.2$
$y = 0.8 - 0.2 = 0.6$
Thus, the overall abundances are $Z^5 = 20\%$, $Z^6 = 20\%$ and $Z^8 = 60\%$. Therefore, all the statements are correct.

Question 49: A

If a metal is more reactive than hydrogen, a displacement reaction will occur resulting in the formation of a salt with the metal cation and hydrogen.

Question 50: B

$6\ FeSO_4 + K_2Cr_2O_7 + 7\ H_2SO_4 \rightarrow 3\ (Fe)_2(SO_4)_3 + Cr_2(SO_4)_3 + K_2SO_4 + 7\ H_2O$
In order to save time, you have to quickly eliminate options (rather than try every combination out).
The quickest way is to do this is algebraically:

For Potassium:
$2b = 2e = 2f$
Therefore, $b = f$.
Option F does not fulfil $b = e = f$.

For Iron:
$a = 2d$
Options C, D and E don't fulfil $a = 2d$.

For Hydrogen:
$2c = 2g$
Therefore, $c = g$.
Option A does not fulfil $c = g$.
This leaves option B as the answer.

Question 51: E

Atoms are electrically neutral. Ions have different numbers of electrons when compared to atoms of the same element. Protons provide just under 50% of an atom's mass, the other 50% is provided by neutrons. Isotopes don't exhibit significantly different kinetics. Protons do indeed repel each other in the nucleus (which is one reason why neutrons are needed: to reduce the electrical charge density).

Question 52: B

The noble gasses are extremely useful, e.g. helium in blimps, neon signs, argon in bulbs. They are colourless and odourless and have no valence electrons. As with the rest of the periodic table, boiling point increases as you progress down the group (because of increased Van der Waals forces). Helium is the most abundant noble gas (and indeed the 2nd most abundant element in the universe).

Question 53: F

This question will discriminate between students who spot short-cuts built into questions to save valuable time and those that simply dive straight in without appraising the question.

The key here is that due to the conservation of energy, all the gravitational potential energy, mgh, at the top of the ramp will be converted to kinetic energy, $\frac{1}{2}mv^2$, at the bottom.
Thus, we can calculate the final velocity using the following: $mgh = \frac{1}{2}mv^2$
Note that the mass cancels so there is no need to use the density and volume information in order to calculate mass. Hence we get: $2gh = v^2$
$V^2 = 2 \times 10 \times 20 = 400$
Therefore, $v = 20\ ms^{-1}$

Question 54: D

Waves do not transfer mass, but their net neutral motions can interfere with each other to cause standing waves or other interference patterns. The energy of a wave depends on frequency, so waves have many different energies. Gamma rays have the highest energy for light, while visible light is lower in energy.

Question 55: A

Multiply by the denominator to give: $(7x + 10) = (3z^2 + 2)(9x + 5)$
Partially expand brackets on right side: $(7x + 10) = 9x(3z^2 + 2) + 5(3z^2 + 2)$
Take x terms across to left side: $7x - 9x(3z^2 + 2) = 5(3z^2 + 2) - 10$
Take x outside the brackets: $x[7 - 9(3z^2 + 2)] = 5(3z^2 + 2) - 10$

Thus: $x = \frac{5(3z^2 + 2) - 10}{7 - 9(3z^2 + 2)}$

Simplify to give: $x = \frac{(15z^2)}{[7 - 9(3z^2 + 2)]}$

Question 56: B

An alpha particle is a helium nucleus consisting of 2 protons and 2 neutrons. An alpha decay therefore reduces the atomic (proton) number by 2 and the mass number by 4. After a single alpha decay, the resulting proton number is 88 and the resulting mass number is 184. As this then splits in to two, the resulting element has a proton number of 44 and a mass number of 92. Gamma radiation does not alter the subatomic particle make-up of an atom.

Question 57: B

The shortest distance between points A and B is a direct line. Using Pythagoras:
The diagonal of a sports field = $\sqrt{40^2 + 30^2} = \sqrt{1{,}600 + 900} = \sqrt{2{,}500} = 50$.
The diagonal between the sports fields = $\sqrt{4^2 + 3^2} = \sqrt{16 + 9} = \sqrt{25} = 5$.
Thus, the shortest distance between A and B = $50 + 5 + 50 = 105\ m$.

Question 58: C

Let $y = 1.25 \times 10^8$; this is not necessary, but helpful, as the question can then be expressed as: $\frac{100y + 10y}{2y} = \frac{110y}{2y} = 55$

Question 59: A

Equate y to give:
$2x - 1 = x^2 - 1$
$\rightarrow x^2 - 2x = 0$
$\rightarrow x(x - 2) = 0$
Thus, x = 2 and x =0
There is no need to substitute back to get the y values as only option A satisfies the x values.

Question 60: B

The ruler and the cruise ship look to be the same size because their edges are in line with Tim's line of sight. His eyes form the apex of two similar triangles. All the sides of two similar triangles are in the same ratio since the angles are the same, therefore:

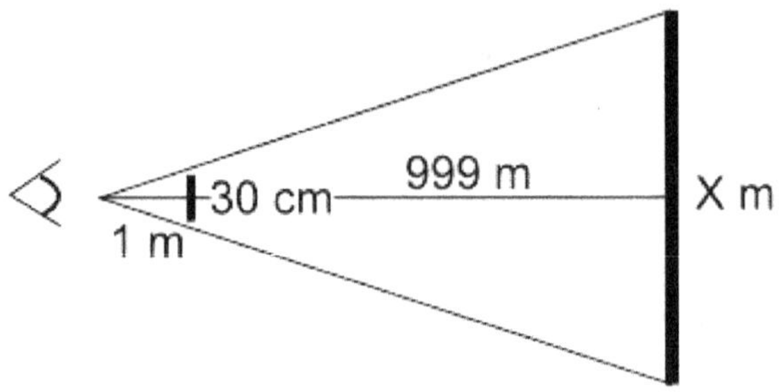

$\frac{0.3m}{X\,m} = \frac{1\,m}{1\,m+999\,m}$

Thus, $X\,m = 1000\,m\,x\,\frac{0.3\,m}{1\,m}$

$1000\,x\,0.3 = 300\,m$

END OF PAPER

Mock Paper G Answers

Question 1: C

B is completely irrelevant to what the manager is saying, so is incorrect. A and E are also incorrect as the manager is simply talking about ticket sales. He has not mentioned anything about the relevant popularity of folk music, or how much the band should value profit. D is incorrect as the manager is simply saying that the band will have higher ticket sales in France than in Germany, so other countries are not relevant. C is correct as Germany could still have higher ticket sales for folk music than France despite the recent changes in ticket sales.

Question 2: E

Ashley has to be sat in the front left seat so there are only two seats left in the front row. Bella and Caitlin have to be sat in different rows, so one of them must be sat in the front row and one in the back row. Now there is only one seat left in the front row, so there is not room for Danielle and her teaching assistant to both sit there. Therefore Danielle and the teaching assistant must take the two remaining seats in the back row. Therefore Emily must sit on the front row as there are no seats remaining in the back row. Emily cannot sit in the middle seat due to her mobility issues, so she must sit in the front right seat.

Question 3: B

Only B is not an assumption, as it is stated in the question that both Grace and Rose departed at 5:15. The other answers are all assumptions. At no point has it been stated that both the girls are walking, or that they will walk at the same speed. If either of these points are incorrect, we cannot definitely state that they will arrive home at the same time. Therefore, A and E are assumptions. Also, it has not been stated that the gymnastics class is being held at the local gymnasium. If this is not the case, then we cannot know how far Grace and Rose have to walk, and therefore cannot state that they will arrive home at the same time. Therefore, C is an assumption. Equally, if Grace gets lost, she may arrive home after Rose, so D is an assumption.

Question 4: D

Let the number of invitations with the extra information in be m. Invitations with extra information in cost £0.70 to send and invitations without cost £0.60. Therefore the total cost of posting is £0.70m + £0.60(50-m) and this is equal to £33. 33=0.70m-0.60m+30. 3=0.1m therefore m=30. So the number of invitations with extra information in is 30. Therefore the answer is D.

Question 5: B

D is irrelevant to the argument's conclusion, whilst A and E are also irrelevant as the argument does not directly imply either of these things (and even if it did they are irrelevant to the argument's conclusions so are not flaws). C is incorrect because the argument states that the Prussian arrival was essential to the British victory, so C is not an assumption. B, however, is never stated in the question, but is needed to be true for the argument's conclusion to be valid.

Question 6: E

A is completely irrelevant to John's conclusions, as the speed of travel has no effect on the train's destination. D is also irrelevant as other destinations from King's Cross station also bear no effect on John's conclusion. Meanwhile, B is incorrect as John's conclusions refer to travelling to Edinburgh by train, so the possibility of travelling by aeroplane has no effect. C is not an assumption because John's conclusion is in the present tense, referring to journeys made at the moment, so future developments have no effect. E is an assumption John has made. Only two other stations in London have been mentioned. At no point has it been mentioned that there are no other stations in London that John could travel from.

Question 7: C

B and D are both stated in the question. A is also stated as the question states that Tanks were a hugely influential factor in ALL battles in World War 2.

E is not stated but is not an assumption as it is not required to be true for the argument's conclusion to be valid.

C however, is required to be true for the conclusion to be valid and yet is never stated in the question, so it is an assumption.

Question 8: E

We can work out the code for each number and see which one equals 3.

The code for A is (3x4) = 12, divided by 6 = 2, minus 1 = 1

The code for B is (9x8) = 72, divided by 6 = 12, minus 4 = 8

The code for C is (5x4) = 20, divided by 2 = 10, minus 3 = 7

The code for D is (7x8) = 56, divided by 4 = 14, minus 8 = 6

The code for E is (6x8) = 48, divided by 4 = 12, minus 9 = 3

Therefore the pin number with the code 3 is E, 6839.

Question 9: E

We can calculate all the rental yields as follows:

House A: (700x12)/168000 = 0.05

House B: (40x125x4)/200000 = 20000/200000 = 0.10

House C: (600*12)/144000 = 7200/144000 = 0.05

House D: (2000*12)/240000 = 24000/240000 = 0.10

House E: (200*52)/100000 = 10400/100000. We can see by observation that this is > 0.1 as 10000/100000 would equal 0.1, therefore there is no need to work this out to be able to say that this is the house with the highest yield.

Question 10: C

The question says that Shaniqua plays in the square which will stop Summer being able to win straight away, so Shaniqua must play in 4. Summer then needs to play in a square where there will be 2 different options to make a line on the turn afterwards, so that Shaniqua cannot block both of them. If Summer plays in 1, she can make a line by playing in either 5 or 6 the next turn, so Shaniqua cannot stop her winning. If Summer plays in 2, she cannot make a line on the next turn at all. If Summer plays in 3, she can only make a line by playing in 6 the next turn and so Shaniqua can stop her. If Summer plays in 5, she can only make a line by playing in 5 the next turn and so Shaniqua can stop her. If Summer plays in 6, she can make a line by playing in either 1 or 3 the next turn, so Shaniqua cannot stop her winning. Therefore she either needs to play in 1 or 6 to be able to be certain of winning the next time.

Question 11: B

A and C can be inferred, as the question states that these things would happen. Meanwhile, D and E actually serve to reinforce the argument's conclusion that the research into a new cure will not be successful. Therefore, they are not flaws in the argument's reasoning.

The point raised by B does weaken the argument and is a valid flaw in the argument's reasoning.

Question 12: B

D and E are both entirely irrelevant to waiting times, so are not flaws.

C is not correct, as the question states that busier ports have longer queuing times. A is also incorrect as the question states that Bordeaux is the busiest port in France, so Calais is definitely less busy than Bordeaux. Therefore, Porto cannot be busier than Bordeaux but less busy than Calais.

B is a flaw, as the fact that Bilbao was busiest last year does not necessarily mean it will be busy this year.

Question 13: B

The volume of the box with 10cm squares cut out is 10*100*100 = 100000cm^3
The volume of the box with 20cm squares cut out is 20*80*80 = 128000cm^3
The volume of the box with 30cm squares cut out is 30*60*60 = 108000cm^3
The volume of the box with 40cm squares cut out is 40*40*40 = 64000cm^3
The volume of the box with 50cm squares cut out is 50*20*20 = 20000cm^3
Therefore the biggest box is the one with the 20cm squares cut out, so the answer is B.

Question 14: A

At no point is A stated, but if aeroplanes are not a major source of carbon dioxide then it does not follow that they are largely responsible for the damage caused by global warming. Therefore, A is a valid assumption.
B and C are both stated in the question, whilst D is irrelevant to the conclusion. E, meanwhile, is stated, as the question states that *we must now seek to curb air traffic in order to save the world's remaining natural environments*.

Question 15: B

B is an underlying assumption in the Transport Minister's argument. If rural areas have plenty of passengers, her assertion that rail companies will not run many services to these areas does not follow from her reasoning. Therefore, if B is true, it strengthens the transport minister's argument.
Meanwhile, D would actually weaken the transport minister's argument, suggesting that privatisation would not lead to less service for rural areas.
C is irrelevant as the transport minister is arguing about how rural communities will be cut off by a privatised system. She is not referring to the quality or price of rail services under a publically subsidised system.
A and E are completely irrelevant points, which have no effect at all on the strength of the Transport Minister's argument.

Question 16: D

At no point does the argument state or imply that we should not be concerned about damage to the polar ice caps, or that reducing energy consumption will not reduce $CO2$ emissions. Therefore, B and E are incorrect.
C could be described as an assumption made in the argument and is therefore not a conclusion.
A goes beyond what the argument says. The argument does not say there are no environmental benefits to reducing energy consumption; it merely says it will not help the Polar Ice Caps. Therefore, A is incorrect and C is a valid conclusion from the argument.

Question 17: B

E is contradictory to the main conclusion of the argument.
A, C and D are all reasons which go on to support the main conclusion of the argument, which is given in B. If we accept A, C and D as true, then it follows readily that the statement given in B is true. Therefore, B is the main conclusion.

Question 18: C

The manager's conclusion (that the centre should hire Candidate 1 in order to maximise profits) relies on the assumption that performance experience, rather than welfare experience, will maximise profits. A valid flaw will mean that this assumption is not valid.

A supports this assumption and so is not a flaw. B is irrelevant as this assumption does not rest on the performance experience being with dolphins specifically. D is irrelevant as it concerns a charity's outlook and is thus not relevant to a profit-making business. If E were indeed a correct prediction then it could still be that profit would rise by *more* with Candidate 1, so the manager may still be correct.
C is a flaw as it expresses a way in which profit may be higher if the business prioritises welfare standards over performance standards, as a boycott of the business could potentially greatly reduce profits.

Question 19: E

A, C and D are all irrelevant to the argument's main conclusion, namely that Egypt was a powerful nation and must therefore have had a very strong military.

B is a conclusion from the argument, but goes on to support E. If a nation required a very strong military to be a powerful nation, then it follows that if Egypt was a powerful nation it must have had a very strong military. Therefore, B is an intermediate conclusion within the argument. E is the *main* conclusion of the argument.

Question 20: C

A), B) and D) are all in direct contradiction to statements made in the passage, so cannot be conclusions. E), meanwhile, does not contradict the argument, but at no point does the argument say that the dangerous isomer was not effective at relieving nausea, so E) is not a conclusion.

However, the fact that the company followed the required level of testing and still did not detect the dangerous isomer does suggest that the required level of testing was not sufficient to identify isomers, so C) is correct.

Question 21: E

General knowledge question

Question 22: B

General knowledge question

Question 23: B

Natural selection favours those who are best suited for survival – this can mean faster and stronger organisms, but not always. For example, snails are pervasive, despite being weak and slow. Variation can arise due to both genetic and environmental components.

Question 24: D

The enzyme amylase catalyses the breakdown of starch into sugars in the mouth (1) and the small intestine (5).

Question 25: E

Whilst there is some enzymatic digestion in 1 and 3, the vast majority occurs in the small intestine (5). The liver facilitates digestion via the production of bile, and the large intestine is primarily responsible for the absorption of water.

Question 26: A

Replotting the genetic diagram with genotype information produces the diagram:

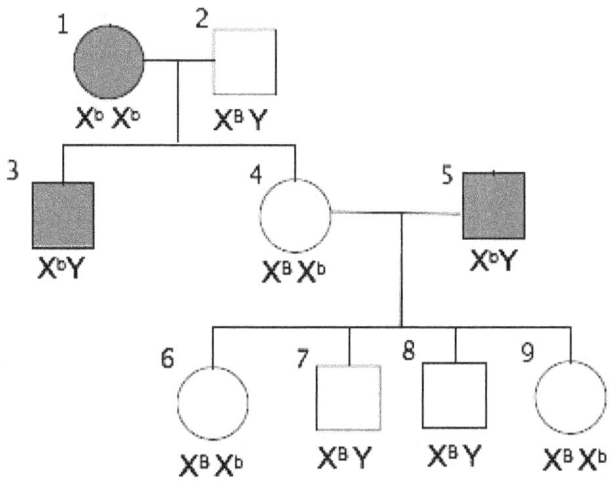

If squares were female, all of 5's circular male offspring would be affected. Circles must be females, so 1 must be homozygous recessive.

Question 27: D

The genotype of a heterozygote female is be $X^B X^b$, and the genotype of 8 is X^B Y. Plotting the information in a Punnett square:

		Female Heterozygote	
		X^B	X^b
Individual 8 (Unaffected Male)	X^B	X^BX^B	X^BX^b
	Y	X^BY	X^bY

The progeny produced are 25% X^BX^B (homozygous normal female), 25% X^BX^b (heterozygous carrier female), 25% X^BY (normal male) and 25% X^bY (affected male). So the chance of producing a colour blind boy is 25%.

Question 28: A

Urine passes from the kidney into the ureter and is then stored in the bladder. It is finally released through the urethra.

Question 29: B

As the known parent has both recessive genotypes, it can only have the gametes, y and t. The next generation has a phenotypic ratio of 1:1:1:1. As both recessive and dominant traits are present in the progeny, the unknown parent's genotype must contain both the recessive and dominant alleles. Hence the unknown parent's genotype must be YyTt as this would produce the gamete combinations of YT, Yt, yT and yt, which when combined with the known yt gametes would result in YyTt, Yytt, yyTt and yytt in equal ratios.

Question 30: D

The possible genotypes are: YYTT (yellow, tall), YyTT (yellow, tall), yyTT (green, tall), YYTt (yellow, tall), YYtt (yellow, short), YyTt (yellow, tall) Yytt (yellow, short), yyTt (green, tall), yytt (green, short). Thus, 9 different genotypes and 4 different phenotypes are possible.

Question 31: D

Whilst getting vitamins, killing bacteria, protein synthesis, and maintaining cellular pH and temperature are all important processes that require a blood supply, the MOST important reason for having a blood supply is the delivery of oxygen and removal of CO_2. This allows aerobic respiration to take place, which produces energy for all of the cell's metabolic processes. None of these processes can be sustained for a meaningful period of time without the energy made available from respiration.

Question 32: A

Insulin works to decrease blood glucose levels. Glucagon causes blood glucose levels to increase; glycogen is a carbohydrate. Adrenaline works to increase heart rate.

Question 33: A

The left side of the heart contains oxygenated blood from the lungs which will be pumped to the body. The right side of the heart contains deoxygenated blood from the body to be pumped to the lungs.

Question 34: A

Since Individual 1 is homozygous normal, and individual 5 is heterozygous and affected, the disease must be dominant. Since males only have one X-chromosome, they cannot be carriers for X-linked conditions. If Nafram syndrome was X-linked, then parents 5 and 6 would produce sons who always have no disease and daughters that always do. As this is not the case shown in individuals 7-10, the disease must be autosomal dominant.

Question 35: C

We know that the inheritance of Nafram syndrome is autosomal dominant, so using N to mean a diseased allele and n to mean a normal allele, 5, 7 and 8 must be Nn because they have an unaffected parent. 2 is also Nn, as if it was NN all its progeny would be Nn and so affected by the disease, which is not the case, as 3 and 4 are unaffected.

Question 36: A

Since 6 is disease free, his genotype must be nn. Thus, neither of 6's parents could be NN, as otherwise 6 would have at least one diseased allele.

Question 37: F

All of the organs listed have endocrine functions. The thyroid produces thyroid hormone. The ovary produces oestrogen. The pancreas secretes glucagon and insulin. The adrenal gland secretes adrenaline. The testes produce testosterone.

Question 38: F

Deoxygenated blood from the body flows through the inferior vena cava to the right atrium where it flows to the right ventricle to be pumped via the pulmonary artery to the lungs where it is oxygenated. It then returns to the heart via the pulmonary vein into the left atrium into the left ventricle where it is pumped to the body via the aorta.

Question 39: E

During inspiration, the pressure in the lungs decreases as the diaphragm contracts, increasing the volume of the lungs. The intercostal muscles contract in inspiration, lifting the rib cage.

Question 40: D

The hypothalamus is the site of central thermoreceptors. A decrease in environmental temperature decreases sweat secretion and causes cutaneous vasoconstriction to minimise heat loss from the blood.

Question 41: H

Chloride is oxidised during this process to form Cl_2. Although the first part of 2) is correct, H_2O is required to dissolve the NaCl (not H_2 which is a product of the reaction). NaOH is a strong base.

Question 42: B

This is an example of an addition reaction, the fluorine and hydrogen atoms are added at the unsaturated bond. If you're unsure about this type of question draw it out and the answer will be obvious.

Question 43: A

The hydrogen halide binds to the alkene's unsaturated double bond. This results in a fully saturated product that consists purely of covalent bonds.

Question 44: F

All of the above are true. Every mole of gas occupies the same volume. The left side therefore occupies 4 volumes, and the right side occupies 2 volumes. Increasing pressure will favour the lower volume side, and the equilibrium will shift right to produce ammonia and decrease the overall volume that the products and reactants occupy. If more N_2 gas is added, equilibrium will shift to react away this gas and lower the concentration again, with the result that more ammonia will be formed.

Question 45: E

Sodium is element 11 on the periodic table, a group 1 element, so has electron configuration: 2, 8, 1. It forms a metallic bond with other sodium atoms. Chlorine is element 17 in group 7, so has 17 electrons and 7 valence electrons, giving configuration: 2, 8, 7. Chlorine forms the covalent gas Cl_2, sharing one electron for a full valence shell.

Salt (NaCl) is an ionic compound, where sodium gives its single valence electron to chlorine so both atoms have full outer electron shells (8 electrons, so 2, 8:2, 8, 8).

Question 46: A

The polymerisation reaction opens the double bond between the two C atoms to allow the formation of a long chain of monomers.

Question 47: C

Assume total mass of molecule is 100g. Therefore, it contains 70.6g carbon, 5.9g hydrogen and 23.5g oxygen. Now, calculate the number of moles of each element using $Moles = \frac{Mass}{Molar\ Mass}$

$$Moles\ of\ Carbon = \frac{70.6}{12} \approx 6$$

$$Moles\ of\ Hydrogen = \frac{5.9}{1} \approx 6$$

$$Moles\ of\ Oxygen = \frac{23.5}{16} \approx 1.5$$

Therefore, the molar ratios give an empirical formula of $C_6H_6O_{1.5} = C_4H_4O$.
Molar mass of the empirical formula = (4 x 12) + (4 x 1) + 16 = 68.
Molar mass of chemical formula = 136. Therefore, the chemical formula = $C_8H_8O_2$.

Question 48: D

Alkenes can be hydrogenated (i.e. reduced) to alkanes. Aromatic compounds are commonly written as cyclic alkenes, but their properties differ from those of alkenes. Therefore alkenes and aromatic compounds do not belong to the same chemical class.

Question 49: A

Transition metals form multiple stable ions which may have many different colours (e.g. green Fe^{2+} and brown Fe^{3+}). They usually form ionic bonds and are commonly used as catalysts (e.g. iron in the Haber process, Nickel in alkene hydrogenation). They are excellent conductors of electricity and are known as the d-block elements.

Question 50: A

The average atomic mass takes the abundances of both isotopes into account:
(Abundance of Cl^{35})(Mass Cl^{35}) + (Abundance of Cl^{37})(Mass Cl^{37}) = 35.453
34.969(Abundance of Cl^{35}) + 36.966(Abundance of Cl^{37}) = 35.453
The abundances of both isotopes = 100% = 1
I.e. abundance of Cl^{35} + abundance of Cl^{37} = 1
Therefore: x + y = 1 which can be rearranged to give: y = 1-x
Therefore: x + (1 – x) = 1.
34.969x + 36.966(1-x) = 35.453
x = 0.758
1 - x = 0.242
Therefore, $Cl^{35}$is 3 times more abundant than Cl^{37}.
Note that you could approximate the values here to arrive at the solution even quicker, e.g. 34.969 → 35, 36.966 → 37 and 35.453 → 35.5

Question 51: B

$2Na + 2H_2O \rightarrow 2NaOH + H_2$
8000 cm^3 = 8 dm^3 = ⅓ moles of H_2
2 moles of Na react completely to form 1 mole of H_2.
Therefore, ⅔ moles of Na must have reacted to produce ⅓ moles of Hydrogen. ⅔ x 23g per mole = 15.3g.
% Purity of sample = $\frac{15.3}{20}$ x 100 = 76.5%

Question 52: B

$S + 6\,HNO_3 \rightarrow H_2SO_4 + 6\,NO_2 + 2\,H_2O$
In order to save time, you have to quickly eliminate options (rather than try every combination out).
The quickest way to do this is algebraically:
For Hydrogen:
b = 2c + 2e
Options A, C, D, E and F don't fulfil b = 2c + 2e.
This leaves options B as the only possible answer.
Note how quickly we were able to get the correct answer here by choosing an element that appears in 3 molecules (as opposed to Sulphur or Nitrogen which only appear in 2).

Question 53: D

The energy in a nuclear bomb comes from $E = mc^2$. When two nuclei fuse, the combined mass is slightly smaller than the two individual nuclei, and the mass lost is converted to energy according to Einstein's equation. Fusion releases much more energy than fission, as in the sun, and humans cannot harness this energy yet. Uncontrolled fission causes the explosion in an atom bomb and is created by a neutron-induced chain reaction. In power plants these neutrons are tightly controlled, so as not to overload the reactors and cause an explosion.

Question 54: B

$$\left(\frac{T}{4\pi}\right)^2 = \frac{l(M+3m)}{3g(M+2m)}$$

$$\frac{T^2}{16\pi^2} x \frac{3g}{l} = \frac{M+3m}{M+2m}$$

$$3gT^2\,(M+2m) = 16l\pi^2(M+3m)$$

$$3gT^2M + 6gT^2m = 16l\pi^2M + 48l\pi^2m$$

$$6gT^2m - 48l\pi^2m = 16l\pi^2M - 3gT^2M$$

$$m(6gT^2 - 48l\pi^2) = 16l\pi^2M - 3gT^2M$$

$$m = \frac{16l\pi^2M - 3gT^2M}{6gT^2 - 48l\pi^2}$$

Question 55: B

The mean is the sum of all the numbers in the set divided by the number of members in the set. The sum of all the numbers in the original set must be: 11 numbers x mean of 6 = 66. The sum of all the numbers once two are removed must then be: 9 numbers x mean of 5 = 45. Thus any two numbers which sum to 66 – 45 = 21 could have been removed from the set.

Question 56: B

R of series circuit= R + R = 2R

R parallel = $\frac{1}{\frac{1}{R}+\frac{1}{R}} = \frac{1}{\frac{2}{R}} = \frac{R}{2}$

Thus, the parallel circuit has a smaller resistance than the series circuit.

Since $I = \frac{V}{R}$, the parallel circuit will have a greater current than the series.

Question 57: B

Let $y = 3.4 \times 10^{10}$; this is not necessary, but helpful, as the question can then be expressed as:

$$\frac{10y + y}{200y} = \frac{11y}{200y} = \frac{11}{200} = \frac{5.5}{100}$$

$$= 5.5 \times 10^{-2}$$

Question 58: E

From the rules of angles made by intersections with parallel lines, all of the angles marked with the same letter are equal. There is no way to find if d = 90°, only that b + d = c = 180° – a = 135°, so b is unknown.

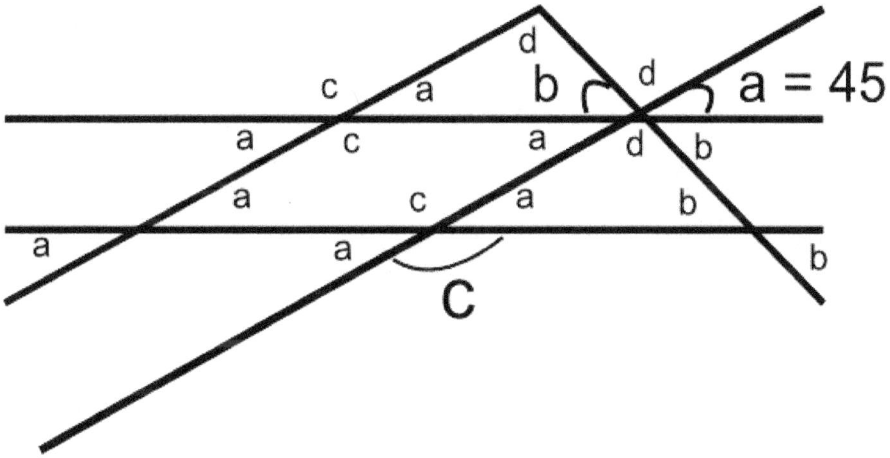

Question 59: B

During electrolysis a current is used to draw charged ions to electrodes. The anode is positively charged and draws anions like sulphate, and the cathode is negatively charged and attracts positively charged cations like copper. For electrolysis to work well, the electrodes need to keep their positive or negative charge. If an alternating AC-current was used, the anode and cathode would repeatedly switch places, and the ions would make no net movement toward either electrode.

Question 60: C

Transform all numbers into fractions then follow the order of operations to simplify. Move the surds next to each other and evaluate systematically:

$$= \left(\left(\frac{6}{8} x \frac{7}{3}\right) \div \left(\frac{7}{5} x \frac{2}{6}\right)\right) x \frac{4}{10} x \frac{15}{100} x \frac{5}{100} x \frac{5}{25} x\ \pi\ x \left(\sqrt{e^2}\right) x\ e\pi^{-1}$$

$$= \left(\frac{42}{24} \div \frac{14}{30}\right) x \frac{4 x 3 x 25}{10 x 20 x 100 x 25} x\ \pi\ x\ \pi^{-1} x\ e^{-1} x\ e$$

$$= \left(\frac{21}{12} \div \frac{7}{15}\right) x \frac{12}{200 x 100} x \frac{\pi}{\pi} x \frac{e}{e}$$

$$= \left(\frac{21}{12} x \frac{15}{7}\right) x \frac{3}{50 x 100}$$

$$= \frac{45}{12} x \frac{3}{5000}$$

$$= \frac{9}{4} x \frac{1}{1000}$$

$$= \frac{9}{4000}$$

END OF PAPER

Mock Paper H Answers

Question 1: A

In this question we are looking at what cannot be reliably concluded from the passage. B and E conclude the state of a substance is not dependent on its chemical properties. C and D discuss how combining two substances can produce a new substance with very different physical properties. The passage refers to how the chemistry of a compound does not necessarily affect the physical properties of that compound. Thus, the answer must be A, which claims the chemical composition of a compound influences its physical nature.

Question 2: C

In this sequence, each alternate letter goes forward starting with B or backwards starting with Y. They start by jumping 4 letters, then 3, then 2 and finally the letters we are trying to find will have jumped by just 1. Thus, the letter after K is L, and the letter before P is O, so the answer is C.

Question 3: E

In this question we are looking at what can be reliably concluded from the passage. The passage is referring to products being made from similar parts; it is the way in which these parts are arranged that actually determines the final product. Thus, B cannot be right. D is also not correct, as there is no mention of protoplasm being the building block for life. E is the correct answer therefore.

Question 4: D

With these questions it is easiest to start at the end of the question and work backwards. The day two days before Monday is Saturday. The day immediately after that is Sunday. The day that comes four days after Sunday is Thursday, and two days after that is Saturday. Thus, the answer is D.

Question 5: D

In this question we are looking at what could weaken the passage above. The passage is discussing synthetic and natural cellulose and how their functions depend on whether the cellulose is plastic or colloidal. However, it states that the properties of natural and synthetic cellulose are equally similar. Therefore, any statement claiming some of the properties between the two forms of cellulose are different would weaken the passage, thus the answer is D.

Question 6: E

In order to work out this question, we need to make some simultaneous equations to relate John and Michael's money. If the amount of money John has at the start is J, and the amount that Michael has is M, we get the following equations:

$J - 20 = 2(M + 20)$ and $J + 5 = 5(M - 5)$, which is simplified to:

$J = 2M + 60$ and $J = 5M - 30$.

Substituting in, to work out M gives:

$2M + 60 = 5M - 30$, thus $3M = 90$ and $M = 30$.

Substituting in $M = 30$ to one of the equations gives:

$J = 60 + 60 = 120$.

Thus, $J + M = 150$, so the answer is E.

Question 7: E

In this question we want a summary of the passage. This passage refers to the use of fire in civilisations to create light. Through the passage it talks about the evolution of the use of fire, finishing with a reference to gas lamps in the street. Thus a good conclusion will refer to how the use of fire has changed over time, but also how lighting one's home is a key factor of civilisation. The answer must therefore be E, which discusses the evolution of fire use and also its importance in civilisation.

Question 8: A

972/2 = 486, thus 486 patients did not have chicken.

972/3 = 324, thus 162 patients did not have the chicken or the mac and cheese.

972/12 = 81, thus 972 – 486 – 324 – 81 = 81, which is the number of patients that had the vegetarian option. Therefore the answer is A.

Question 9: C

In this question we are looking at what can be reliably concluded from the passage. The passage does not tell us exactly how phosphorous was discovered, but we know that it was not Wilhelm Homberg who discovered it, thus A, B and D cannot be correct. 1669 is not in the 18th century thus E is also false. The passage describes how the element phosphorous was discovered by accident, by a man of low social status. Therefore, C is the only correct answer.

Question 10: D

For this question refer to the times in minutes, rather than hours, so 3pm is 180 minutes. x is the number of minutes past noon that we are trying to find. Therefore x + 28 will give the same amount of minutes past noon as 180-3x.

$x + 28 = 180 - 3x$

$4x = 152$

x = 38, thus the answer is D.

Question 11: B

In this question we are trying to find a suitable conclusion to the passage. A and E are completely irrelevant to the passage. C is incorrect as wings only attach to the posterior two segments of the insect's body. While D is correct, the legs are not referenced as being the most important part of the insect's body. Thus the answer must be B, which states the wings are the most dominant part of the body.

Question 12: D

For John: 56/64 x 100 = 87.5% or 7/8

For Mary: 24/36 x 100 = 66.7% or 2/3

Therefore we need to work out 7/8 – 2/3

21/24 – 16/24 = 5/24. Multiply by 100 to get the actual percentage:

500/24 = 125/6, thus the answer is D.

Question 13: A

To calculate this one needs to find the lowest common multiple of both 73 and 104, and then add that value to 2007. The lowest common multiple of 73 and 104 is 7592, which when added to 2007 gives 9559AD.

Question 14: B

If the number of girls is 40 more than the number of boys, and the boys make up 40% of the total number of students, then the discrepancy of 40 between boys and girls must represent 20%. Therefore, 1%=2 students and therefore the total number of students is 200.

Question 15: C

Based on the information, the school bus will get her to school at 09:01. The public bus arrives at 08:21, which she will miss, and the next bus will arrive at 08:38, which will take 18 minutes to arrive, meaning she will at school at 08:56, so the public bus at 08:38 will get her to school first.

Question 16: B

In this question we want a summary of the passage. The passage talks mostly about the feeding habits of the puddle duck, thus a summary discussing the predation of puddle ducks is irrelevant, meaning A and D are not correct. E is wrong as puddle ducks mainly live in shallow waters, and this is not because of their eating habits so C is also wrong. Thus, B is the correct answer as the ducks feed on mainly vegetarian food sources, and although they can dive for food, this is not their main route of feeding.

Question 17: A

In this question we want a summary of the passage. The veil discussed is clearly involved in a connection between the good and evil of the earth and therefore of mankind. Thus for a good summarising sentence, we want this connection to be discussed. Therefore, the answer must be A, which states that the veil links the good and evil of the human race, as is discussed in the passage.

Question 18: E

There is a specific sequence linking these numbers. Multiplying the first and third numbers of each row gives a number that makes up the second and fourth numbers of the same row.
9 x 3 = 27, thus the missing number is 7 and the answer is E.

Question 19: C

In this question we are looking to find the flaw in the argument. Answers D and E are irrelevant to the question. While B is correct it does not explain why the metformin inhibitor would have not had any effect on metformin's inhibition of fat cell growth. The key problem here is we are not given any information about the metformin inhibitor mentioned, and thus are not able to judge how it would affect metformin's fat cell growth inhibition, thus the answer is C.

Question 20: C

We do not know whether Alexandra and Katie are dancers, so **A** and **B** are wrong. We do not know whether any dancers are ugly, so **D** is wrong.

Question 21: D

General knowledge question

Question 22: A

General knowledge question

Question 23: A

HCO_3^- is an alkaline substance and a vital component of the physiological buffering system. If the pH of the blood drops below 7, the bicarbonate molecule will accept a H^+ whereas if the pH increase, it will release H^+, thus HCO_3^- is an alkali.

Question 24: D

The diaphragm is crucial to breathing as during inhalation it contracts and expands the chest space, along with the intercostal muscles which draw the ribs upwards and outwards, effectively lowering the pressure within the thoracic cavity and drawing air into the lungs. During exhalation all the muscles relax which lets the ribs drop downwards and inwards and the diaphragm balloons upwards into the chest space. This increases the pressure within the thoracic cavity which forces air out of the lungs.

Question 25: E

Some students may think that the arteries carry oxygenated blood from the mother to the foetus and that the vein carries the deoxygenated blood from the foetus to the mother, but it is important to remember that arteries always carry blood to the heart (in this case the mother's) and veins always travel away from the heart. A prime example of this is the pulmonary system, as like the foetal-mother system, the pulmonary arteries carry deoxygenated blood to the lungs away from the heart and the pulmonary veins carry oxygenated blood back to the heart.

Question 26: H

The kidneys are involved in ultrafiltration as they filter all of the blood in the body of toxins/waste products from metabolic reactions. The waste is released as urine via the bladder. Some of the water is filtered out then reabsorbed by the kidney, especially when the body is dehydrated. Although glucose is reabsorbed by the kidney, it does not play a part in glucose regulation as that is mainly done by the pancreas by secretion of insulin and glucagon. These hormones are two of many found in the body, none of which are produced by the kidneys. There are some that are produced by the adrenal cortices that sit atop the kidneys, but these are a separate anatomical structure from the kidney.

Question 27: A

Haemophilia B is an X-linked recessive disorder which means you need two copies of the faulty genes in girls to present the phenotype associated with the disease and only one copy in males as they have XY chromosomes and are thus missing the extra X chromosome which may have carried the healthy, dominant gene. As Mike, the father of the baby girl, is not affected, we can assume that the mother carries one copy of the faulty gene herself. Thus, although the baby girl will not be affected by the condition, she may be a carrier of the gene and so, can pass it on to future generations.

Question 28: F

The first line defence of the body from invading pathogens is the skin. This is a tough keratinized layer, which is not easily broken down by bacteria. There is also flora on the skin (bacteria that live on the skin) that prevents any harmful bacteria from colonising. The next line of defence is the mucus lining the airways. It traps dirt and pathogens, to be either expelled from the body or swallowed into the gut. The next layer of defence mentioned in the answers, is hydrochloric acid found in the stomach. This has a pH of 2 and so effectively kills any pathogens that enter the body through the food. Other defences not listed include, tears (they contain lysozymes that break down the bacteria) and acidic substances by the sebaceous glands of the skin.

Some students may get confused by the antibodies. Although it is true that antibodies provide a line of defence, they are a secondary line of defence after the pathogen has got past the initial defences.

Question 29: C

Osmosis is the movement of water particles across a partially permeable membrane from an area of low concentration to an area of high concentration (of solute). It is not an active process as water can easily diffuse through bilipid layer membranes and thus does not require a specific passage.

Question 30: B

Plants also give off carbon via respiration and death. Although some of the carbon is given off, trees and plants do store carbon in their cells and thus they are known as carbon stores.

Question 31: A

Enzymes are always substrate specific as the active site is made up of a specific set of amino acids that determine which reaction the enzyme catalyses.

Question 32: D

Whilst A, B, C and E are true of the DNA code, they do not represent the property described, which is that more than one combination of codons can encode the same amino acid, e.g. Serine is coded by the sequences: TCT, TCC, TCA, TCG.

Question 33: B

The degenerate nature of the code can help to reduce the deleterious effects of point mutations. The several 3-nucleotide combinations that code for each amino acid are usually similar such that a point mutation, i.e. a substitution of one nucleotide for another, can still result in the same amino acid as the one coded for by the original sequence.

Question 34: A

The movement of carbon dioxide in the lungs and neurotransmitters in a synapse are both examples of diffusion. Glucose reabsorption is an active process, as it requires work to be done against a concentration gradient.

Question 35: F

Some enzymes contain other molecules besides protein, e.g. metal ions. Enzymes can increase rates of reaction that may result in heat gain/loss, depending on if the reaction is exothermic or endothermic. They are prone to variations in pH and are highly specific to their individual substrate.

Questions 36: E

Statements 1 and 3 are correct. Statement 2 in incorrect, as it is the 4 carbon molecule oxaloacetate that is regenerated. Oxaloacetate combines with acetyl CoA to form the 6 carbon citrate.

Question 37: B

Statement 1 and 3 are incorrect. Cyclic phosphorylation doesn't require water as no photolysis occurs, the electrons are just passed back to the chlorophyll molecule. Photolysis only occurs in PSII, because this is where the enzymes are. Statement 2 is correct, photolysis of water produces protons, which can reduce NADP.

Question 38: C

Statement 1 is incorrect as RUBISCO is an enzyme that fixes carbon dioxide to RuBP. Statement 2 is correct. 6 turns of the cyle produce 12 triose phosphate moleucles. 10 are used to regenerate RuBP, and 2 removed from the cycle to form one molecule of glucose

Question 39: F

Statement 1 is correct, sodium ions drive depolarisation and potassium ions drive repolarisation. Statement 2 is correct, as hyperpolarisation prevents the initiation of another action potential in the region that has just been depolarised, so the action potential can only travel forwards. Statement 3 is correct. As temperature increases action potentials travel faster, up to around 40°C after which the proteins start to denature. Larger diameter axons have less electrical resistance, so action potentials can travel faster.

Question 40: E

Statement 1 is correct, if too much insulin is given then the blood glucose level can fall dangerously low. Statement 2 in incorrect, adrenaline increased blood glucose to allow the body to respond to a fight-or-flight situation. Statement 3 is correct, glucagon causes glycogen to be hydrolysed into glucose (glycogenolysis), and fatty acids and amino acids to be converted into glucose (gluconeogenesis)

Question 41: C

ΔH is positive because the enthalpy of the products is higher than the enthalpy of the reactants. This also means that the reactants are less stable than the products and because it is ENDOthermic, energy is absorbed from the surroundings.

Question 42: A

There are several methods to work this out, one of which is shown below.

Mass of FeS_2 in the ore = 480 x 0.75 = 360kg

1 mole of FeS_2 = 55 + 32 + 32 = 119g → this can be rounded to 120g for ease of calculation.

Number of moles of FeS_2 in the ore = $\frac{360 \times 10^3}{120} = 3 \times 10^3$ mol

Mass of Fe = $(3 \times 10^3) \times 55$ = 165kg.

167.7kg is closest to this value.

Question 43: B

Here, it is important to remember the reactivity series.

This is important as it tells you which elements are able to displace other elements in redox reactions. In this example, Zinc is the only element above Iron in the series and thus, is the only element that would be able to displace Iron.

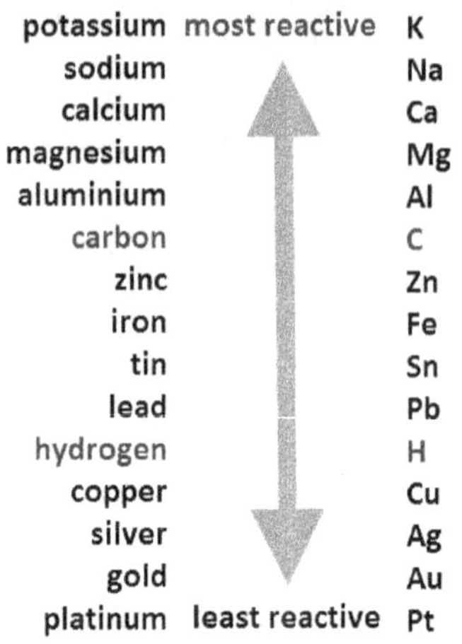

Question 44: A

Catalysts increase the rate of reaction by providing an alternative reaction path with a lower activation energy, which means that less energy is required and so costs are reduced. The point of equilibrium, the nature of the products, and the overall energy change are unaffected by catalysts.

Question 45: A

In the diagram shown, the number at the top (73) denotes the mass number of an atom of Germanium. This is the number of protons and neutrons in the nucleus. The number at the bottom (32) is the proton number, i.e. the number of protons in the nucleus. Protons have a positive charge, neutrons have a neutral charge and electrons have a negative charge. As a stable element, Germanium must have a charge of 0 and thus the electrons and protons have to cancel out. Therefore, Germanium has 32 electrons.

Question 46: A

This is complete combustion as all of the methane is used to make water and carbon dioxide. It is an aerobic reaction as oxygen is present and needed to cause the combustion of the fuel. By increasing the carbon dioxide in the system you would either slow down or not affect the rate of combustion, but definitely would not speed it up. This also applies to removing oxygen from the system.

Question 47: A

Alkenes undergo addition reactions, such as that with hydrogen, when catalysed by nickel, whilst alkanes do not as they are already fully saturated. The C=C bond is stronger than the C-C bond, but it is not exactly twice as strong, so will not require twice the energy to break it. Both molecules are organic and will dissolve in organic solvents.

Question 48: F

Diamond is unable to conduct electricity because all the electrons are involved in covalent bonds. Graphite is insoluble in water + organic solvents. Graphite is also able to conduct electricity because there are free electrons that are not involved in covalent bonds.

Methane and Ammonia both have low melting points. Methane is not a polar molecule, so cannot conduct electricity or dissolve in water. Ammonia is polar and will dissolve in water. It can conduct electricity in aqueous form, but not as a gas.

Question 49: E

The 5 carbon atoms in this hydrocarbon make it a "pent" stem. The C=C bond makes it an alkene, and the location of this bond is the 2nd position, making the molecule pent-2-ene.

Question 50: D

Group 1 elements form positively charged ions in most reactions and therefore lose electrons. Thus, the oxidation number must increase. Their reactivity increases as the valence electrons are further away from the positively charged nucleus down group. All group one elements react spontaneously with oxygen – the less reactive ones form an oxide coating and the more reactive ones spontaneously burn.

Question 51: H

The cathode attracts positively charged ions. The cathode reduces ions and the anode oxidises ions. Electrolysis can be used to separate compounds but not mixtures (i.e. substances that are not chemically joined).

Question 52: B

Pentane, C_5H_{12}, has a total of 3 isomers. A, C and D are correctly configured. However, the 4th Carbon atom in option B has more than 4 bonds which wouldn't be possible. If you're stuck on this – draw them out!

Question 53: B

The current in a series circuit is always the same at any point in the circuit according to Kirchoff's first law which states that *at any node or junction in a circuit the sum of the current flowing into that node is equal to the current leaving that same node.* Thus current is always conserved. Since a series circuit does not have any nodes or junctions, we can assume the current is constant throughout.

The potential difference is shared between all the components of the circuit ($V_{total} = V_1 + V_2 + V_3...$). This is because the total work done on the charge by the battery must equal the total work done by the charge on the components.

Resistance in a series circuit is the sum of all the individual resistances (R = R1 + R2 + R3…). The resistance of two or more resistors is bigger than the resistance of just one of the resistors on its own because the battery has to push charge through all of them.

Question 54: B

There are several steps to solving this problem. The first is to work out the area of the entire floor, minus the fish tank and the cut out corner. We can see that the length of the room is 8m and the width of the room is 4m (the sides of the cut out square are 2m). Thus the area of the entire room is **32m²**.

The cut out corner is a square with the dimension 2 x 2m. Thus the area of the cut out corner is **4m²**.

The fish tank is a circle, so its area will be πr^2. Π is taken to be 3 and thus $3 \times 1^2 =$ **3m²**.

Therefore the floor area, Bill needs to cover is 32 – (4 + 3) = ***25m²***.

We then need to work out the area of one plank. The dimensions of this are in cm and so we need to convert to m. 1m is 100cm and so we can say that the length of the plank is 0.6m and the width is 0.1m. Thus the area is 0.6 x 0.1 = ***0.06m²***.

To work out the number of planks, required, we need to divide the area of the floor space by the area of the plank. A quick way of doing this would be rounding the area of the room down to 24 and multiplying the area of the plank by 100 so it becomes 6.

24/6 = 4, then because we multiplied the area of the plank by 100, we then multiply the answer by 100 which gives us ***400 planks.*** The closest answer to our solution is 417, which is listed as B.

Question 55: B

Solve $y = x^2 - 3x + 4$ and $y - x = 1$ as (x,y).

Substitute the quadratic expression into the other non-quadratic. You'll get another equation.

$x + 1 = x^2 - 3x + 4$

Rearrange to get a quadratic equation and solve.

$x^2 - 4x + 3 = 0$

$(x - 1)(x - 3) = 0$

Therefore $x = 1$ or $x = 3$

Substitute your x values into the equation, $y - x = 1$ and solve to work out y values.

$y = 2$ or $y = 4$

Therefore the coordinates are (1, 2) and (3, 4)

Question 56: A

The gravitational potential energy of the ball at the top of the slope is *mgh*. The kinetic energy of the ball as it travels down the slope is $0.5mv^2$. The gravitational potential energy = kinetic energy, therefore:

$mgh = 0.5mv^2$

The mass values on either side cancel out to leave: $gh = 0.5v^2$

Thus we can substitute values into the equation:

$10 \times 5 = 0.5 \times v^2$

$50 = 0.5 \times v^2$

$50/0.5 = v^2$

$\sqrt{100} = v = 10$

Question 57: A

As galaxies and celestial objects move away from Earth, the wavelength of the light they emit, gets longer as it travels towards us. Thus there is a noticeable shift towards the red end of the spectrum, when we measure those waves. Scientists are able to measure the real light coming from galaxies far away using telescopes that pick up and record this light. Using red shift we can tell which galaxies are further away and which ones are closer. There is another phenomena called blue shift, which is the opposite of red shift in that, we can tell which galaxies are moving closer to us as the wavelengths of those galaxies become shorter and therefore shift to the blue end of the spectrum.

Question 58: A

X-rays are able to pass through soft, less dense material, like skin, soft tissue and air to stain the x-ray film black. They can't pass through denser material like bone and thus the x-ray film stays white. X-rays are harmful with prolonged exposure as they ionise cells and cause DNA damage that can result in conditions like cancer. Radiologists or technicians working with x-rays wear lead aprons to protect them from excess radiation. Gamma rays are different to x-rays with shorter wavelengths that are able to pass through dense material and because of this, they are considered more dangerous than x-rays.

Question 59: A

$\frac{(16x+11)}{(4x+5)} = 4y^2 + 2$

$16x + 11 = (4y^2 + 2)(4x + 5)$

$16x + 11 = 4x(4y^2 + 2) + 5(4y^2 + 2)$

$16x - 4x(4y^2 + 2) = 5(4y^2 + 2) - 11$

$x(16 - 4(4y^2 + 2) = 20y^2 - 1$

$X = \frac{20y^2-1}{[16-4(4y^2+2)]}$

Question 60: D

The first step is to multiply out $(3p + 5)^2$

$(3p + 5)(3p + 5) = 24p + 49$

$9p^2 + 30p + 25 = 24p + 49$

$9p^2 + 6p - 24 = 0$

Then put the quadratic into brackets.

$(3p + 6)(3p - 4) = 0$

Therefore p must equal -6 or +4.

END OF PAPER

FINAL ADVICE

Arrive well rested, well fed and well hydrated

The IMAT is an intensive test, so make sure you're ready for it. Unlike the UKCAT, you'll have to sit this at a fixed time (normally at 9AM). Thus, ensure you get a good night's sleep before the exam (there is little point cramming) and don't miss breakfast. If you're taking water into the exam then make sure you've been to the toilet before so you don't have to leave during the exam. Make sure you're well rested and fed in order to be at your best!

Move on

If you're struggling, move on. Every question has equal weighting and there is no negative marking. In the time it takes to answer on hard question, you could gain three times the marks by answering the easier ones. Be smart to score points- especially in section two where some questions are far easier than others.

Make Notes on your Essay

Some universities may ask you questions on your IMAT essay at the interview. Sometimes you may have the interview as late as March which means that you **MUST** make short notes on the essay title and your main arguments after the essay. This is especially important if you're applying to UCL and Cambridge where the essay is discussed more frequently.

Afterword

Remember that the route to a high score is your approach and practice. Don't fall into the trap that "*you can't prepare for the IMAT*"– this could not be further from the truth. With knowledge of the test, some useful time-saving techniques and plenty of practice you can dramatically boost your score.

Work hard, never give up and do yourself justice.

Good Luck!

Acknowledgements

I would like to thank the UniAdmissions Tutors for all their hard work and advice in compiling this book.

Alex

About Us

Infinity Books is the publishing division of *Infinity Education Ltd.* We currently publish over 85 titles across a range of subject areas – covering specialised admissions tests, examination techniques, personal statement guides, plus everything else you need to improve your chances of getting on to competitive courses such as medicine and law, as well as into universities such as Oxford and Cambridge.

Outside of publishing we also operate a highly successful tuition division, called UniAdmissions. This company was founded in 2013 by Dr Rohan Agarwal and Dr David Salt, both Cambridge Medical graduates with several years of tutoring experience. Since then, every year, hundreds of applicants and schools work with us on our programmes. Through the programmes we offer, we deliver expert tuition, exclusive course places, online courses, best-selling textbooks and much more.

With a team of over 1,000 Oxbridge tutors and a proven track record, UniAdmissions have quickly become the UK's number one admissions company.

Visit and engage with us at:

Website (Infinity Books): www.infinitybooks.co.uk

Website (UniAdmissions): www.uniadmissions.co.uk

Facebook: www.facebook.com/uniadmissionsuk

Twitter: @infinitybooks7

www.ingramcontent.com/pod-product-compliance
Lightning Source LLC
Chambersburg PA
CBHW081153290426
44108CB00018B/2537
* 9 7 8 1 9 1 2 5 5 7 8 1 3 *